Ulrich Klever

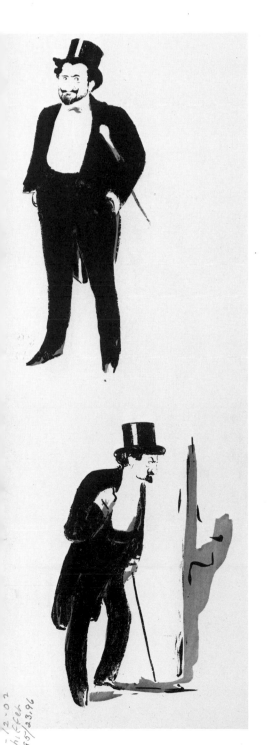

Walkingsticks

Accessory, tool and symbol

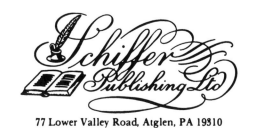
Schiffer Publishing Ltd

77 Lower Valley Road, Atglen, PA 19310

Dedicated to my daughter Katrin and my son-in-law Dr. Hans-Joachim Schubert —
diligent helpers in my collecting

The canes shown in the illustrations are from German, Swiss, English and French private collections, unless otherwise indicated. In accordance with the owners' wishes, they remain anonymous. I wish to thank every one of them for their cooperation. Everyone of them has served the "Cane Affair" tremendously.

Fig. 1 Monsieur Galland and his cane. Double sheet lithograph by SEM (= Georges Goursat 1863-1934).

Library of Congress Cataloging-in-Publication Data

Klever, Ulrich, 1922-
[Spazierstöcke. English]
Walkingsticks : accessory, tool, and symbol / Ulrich Klever.
p.   cm.
Includes bibliographical references and index.
ISBN 0-7643-0013-X (pbk.)
1. Staffs (Sticks, canes, etc.) I. Title.
GT2220.K5513   1996
391'.44--dc20   96-29305
                                 CIP

Published by Schiffer Publishing, Ltd.
77 Lower Valley Road
Atglen, PA 19310
(610) 593-1777
Fax: (610) 593-2002
Please write for a free catalog.
This book may be purchased from the publisher.
Please include $2.95 for shipping.
Try your bookstore first.

We are interested in hearing from
authors with book ideas on related subjects.

Contents

Contents

Introduction

When the world was full of canes

A whole book about canes? A book on this elongated object, which, according to the dictionary, "is taken on walks, in order to facilitate walking."

What associations do we make with the term "cane?" Initially probably the walking aide, the third leg, the ebony cane with a silver knob which, in memory, grandfather has leaning in the wardrobe. Then, of course, there is the typical German walking stick, which is purchased on vacation, decorated with cane nails and brought home as a souvenir. Its decoration, vanity and actual uselessness is what makes the walking stick a strolling stick. Maybe we also think of the cane of the Old Fritz (Frederick the Great), which combines all the characteristics of a cane. His cane's primary function was as a walking aide, which we can see on numerous prints; its secondary function was as a tool and emblem of power: the King frequently would hit slow servants, exhausted soldiers and lazy administrators. Finally, it had a symbolic function — the cane with the slightly curved handle was part of the Old Fritz, which to this day in German is called a "Fritz handle."

Until 10 years ago I did not have any other associations with canes myself. One day I received three canes as a present, unusual objects and not what I had so far considered as canes. The first has a black agate ball, cut as an ox eye on a honey colored, flexible Malacca cane shaft. The provenance of this cane was known to me: for 50 years it had accompanied its owner and then it had sat in a corner for another 30 years. An everyday story.

The second cane could tell its history (illustr. 46). An anonymous farmer somewhere in Europe had told his story in hard wood. He carved himself, his father, and his dog catching a bird. A large fish lies with the fishing rod next to it. Some chickens run around his house and a cow ruminates. Also found on the cane are very realistic pair of boots, some plants, baskets, a bowl, a book and the most beautiful image of the knife which had been used to carve this cane. I own several of these story canes.

The third cane was one to dream about. It had a handle with integrated opera glasses and a whistle. Which theater scandals was it part of; maybe it started its career at the Opera Comique in Paris on March 3, 1875, witnessing the flop of Carmen.

These three canes started a collection, and if one collects something one wants to know more about ones objects of desire. What kinds of canes exist? How long have they existed? Who made them? Who sold them? Who wore them? How were they worn?

Which woods were used? Which other materials? Besides mass produced canes, were doubles made? Never any? Question after question, and collecting makes one curious.

I started researching. I studied prints with a cane collector's eyes. I looked through old newspapers for notes on canes. And the canes found me.

In 1980, I published my first small German guide book on canes. Now I present this more elaborate book, which is an attempt to show walking and strolling canes in their multitudes. To put them in order by period and mode, to show their use and to reveal their production techniques. This is only a small portion of the cultural history of canes, which begins with the cane of the pharaoh, and continues on in so many forms: the cane as a means of punishment, as a symbol of the guilds, as the scepter of rulers and sign of power for bishops, its importance in heraldry and as an attribute for saints. The entire cane and stick subject is too broad to be dealt with in depth.

The history of the cane started during the uncertain times of the Thirty Years War, when gentlemen were dressed as if they were Wallenstein's brutal soldiers. Around 1630 Monsieur Alamodo also bought a walking and strolling cane. At about the same time, that cane is described and illustrated in German loose letters (see fig. 13) and in English anti-fashion pamphlets. Until 1750 the man of the world carried both a sword and a cane at the same time; after that the sword was taken off, and only the cane was omnipresent until 1930. The cane was part of the outfit; it was adapted to fashion trends or dictated them.

Everybody carried one — there are children's canes, lady's canes, gentlemen's canes, tail coat canes, weapon canes, and professional canes, mass produced products and unique pieces, inventor's canes and family heirlooms, simple canes, artistic canes, and pompous canes. Either used as a functional every day piece or as an aesthetic attribute, the cane underscored ones personality and was used for flirting, discussing or strolling. Let us bring it to this common denominator: the most important purpose of the cane was to put something into a man's hand.

The briefcase together with the bicycle, and later the car, swiftly extinguished the cane's life. Unless a cane fulfills a special purpose as a crutch for the sick or as a walking stick vacation accessory, nobody needs a cane. Their hands are full and they have no spare time.

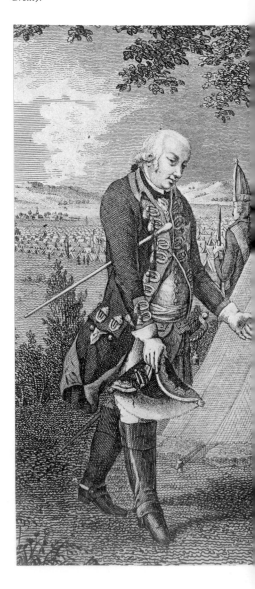

Fig. 2 Various methods to wear one's cane. Copper etching by F. Calau, 1802, from a series about Friedrich den Grossen (Frederick the Great).

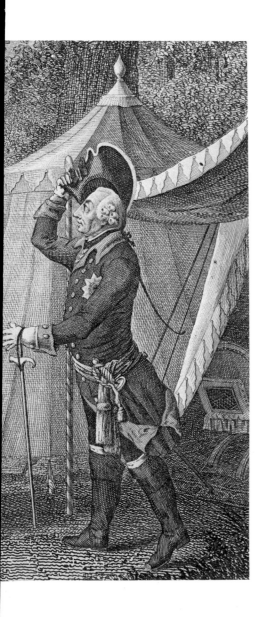

A cane needs time, it inspires its carrier to go for walks, to strolling without purpose. And the cane also needs attention; in its truest sense, walking elegantly with a cane is an art which has to be learned.

When in 1980 the exhibition "Le monde inconnu des cannes" ("The unknown world of canes") opened, the press coverage spread world wide. The reporters were full of nostalgia for what they had seen: canes made of whale bones, glass, paper discs, rhinoceros skin and malacca; handles in silver, ivory and horn; handles fashioned as dog's heads, skulls, hands, ladies legs, sprawling lions and balls which could be opened and contained compasses, dice and lighters. It is almost unbelievable what cane makers and their patrons came up with.

With a few exceptions, the illustrated canes presented here are from private collections, owned by people who share my passion. I would like to thank all of them, they saved many canes from extinction and they made this book about this useful ... and useless ... article possible.

In the world of museums and art historians, the canes always remained a step child. Our museum is this book. Maybe it will inspire you to collect canes. It is interesting to look at canes and there is a special appeal in touching canes. To be able to hold and study canes at the same time is wonderful.

Weisham Estate, in the spring of 1984

Ulrich Klever

Literature about the cane has been sparse. Books that deal with fashion usually do not mention the cane, forget about it, or mention it with a few lines, such as "another fashionable attribute is the cane, which we saw carried by the Alamode cavaliers by the beginning of the century." In memoirs, private correspondence and period writings we can find them mentioned, as in the "memoirs of the Count de Saint Simon" from the court of Louis XIV, the scene in Marly 1695. The King witnessed a servant taking a waffle from the table and putting it into his pocket. "In this moment the King forgets about his dignity, and, cane in hand, which had been just handed to him together with his hat, he ran toward the servant, surprising all around him and hit and cursed at the servant and broke the cane on his back. It had been only a thin cane though." Or the description of a fashionable man in the memoirs of the Marquise of Crequi just before the French revolution in 1789: "The hairstyle a la debacle (a disaster) with a short pony tail without net and 7 or 8 ounces of powder on the collar and the back. Two long watch chains, with numerous hollow acorns, small bells and other curiosities as fobs. To complete this outfit one would wear a little cane in hand made of flexible material, similar to the ones used by servants to dust the upholstery."

This kind of research requires a lot of reading and a filing cabinet. A similar effort must be made to read periodicals in a systematic way. My finds in "Journal des Luxus und der Moden" and in the "Gartenlaube" and "Leipziger Illustrierte Zeitung" will be presented at a later point. Researching the illustrated magazines of the 19th century would be a wonderful task for a future canes researcher.

The magazines of the turners' and cane makers' trade are a good source of information, as are catalogues of cane manufactories, ware houses and mail order catalogues, providing individual pieces of a puzzle which can then be put together. Most informative are illustrations, painting or prints, lithographs and drawings. These portraits, genre scenes, and illustrations often show canes and one can draw one's own conclusion. An example is F.W. Koebner's article for "The Gentlemen," 1913. In "The Gentleman" he (together with other authors) describes how from hat to shirt, from monocle to proper greeting, the "man of world manages the decorations of his life." The cane is mentioned only briefly in the text, no chapter is devoted to it.

But, every single illustration shows the gentleman wearing his cane, and in many different ways. Was the cane so normal that

How to write cane history

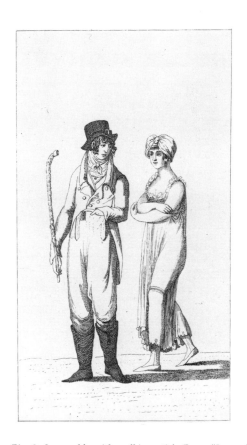

Fig. 3 Incroyable with walking stick. From "Journal des Luxus under der Moden," 1800. (see also text on page 24).

it was not worth mentioning? It is left to the present day author to draw conclusions, put pieces together and voice and opinion.

In articles about canes, published after 1928, Max von Boehn is the dominant figure, and is either cited or provides the basic information. The chapter "The cane" in his book "Beiwerk der Mode" is the most in depth social history of the subject and the most often used source. In addition, the book is not rare and after the war was translated into English. Some articles on canes are simple short versions of von Boehn's book, and the most persistent is his wrong citation from de la Salle: "J.B. de la Salle, who in 1782 published his etiquette, gives numerous instructions. One is not supposed to take a cane to noble people. It is improper to fiddle with it; or to touch someone with it; or to pretend to hit somebody would be the climax of bad taste. One is not allowed to hold it under the arm or to lean on it while standing, to write in the sand with it while sitting, or to pull it behind while walking." Besides the fact, that period prints very well show gentlemen with thin canes under the arm or leaning against canes, I have found differences while studying the original text. The doctor of theology J.B. de la Salle published the book "Les Regles de la Bienseance et de la Civilite Chretienne" in 1840 in Lille. The book about etiquette deals with proper behavior, body care and Christian life style. The cane is mentioned only once: "While walking one should carry the cane in hand, upright against the body, not pressing against it, but loose and neither should shake the cane, the muff, nor the gloves, nor should one carry it with both hands in front of the torso or stomach."

Cane and staff: special symbols

Beginning in ancient history the terms cane and staff are distinguished: The cane has a helping, punishing or decorative function; the staff is a symbol of dignity, authority and power.

In other cultures they were carried by gods, when they were still visible to human beings: Zeus had a staff, Poseidon had a trident, Dionysious had a long Thyros staff, decorated with vines with an ivy or pine cone tip. Asklepios from Epidauros had his staff, with a serpent winding upwards. In Rome this healing god was called Askulap. The nordic god Odin/Wotan also wore a cane/spear, while Donar/Thor carried a long shafted hammer made from the wood of an ash tree. And what was done by gods was carried on by the priests: they also stressed their positions by carrying staffs.

The golden Tutankhamen was a cane lover, and one could call him the first cane collector. His researcher Howard Carter writes: "The young Tutankhamen must have been a lover and collector of canes and staffs, because we found a large number of them in the grave chamber." They were applied with metal, colorful barks and glass, decorated with feathers and shining beetle wings or animal ornaments. They were usually made of hard woods and covered with hieroglyphs. The upper end sometimes had a handle. A large monograph has been written about the canes of the pharaohs.

The Israelis carried plain shepherd's staffs. They called these staffs kanch, which is also a measure for length. The French term canne is also a measure, its German equivalent the "Rohr-Elle," which is 2.23 meters. In the Old Testament no cane is mentioned more than the one of Moses. With the cane Moses and his brother Aaron bring the plagues over Egypt. Water is converted into blood with the blow of that cane, the mosquitos come out of the cane and the cane pointed toward heaven brings thunder and hale and the winds, which will carry the grasshoppers.

The most intriguing for the cane collector is the snake cult. The Egyptian magicians carried snake canes, which ended in the image of a uraeus snake, which belongs to the family of cobras. They could bring those canes to life at will.

According to the 2nd book of the Bible, Moses and Aaron threw the cane in front of the pharaoh and his men and the cane turned

Tutankhamen's grave and the cane cult of the Israelis

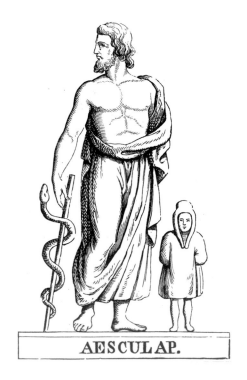

AESCULAP.

Fig. 4 Woodcut "The Olymp" by A.H. Petiscus, Leipzig, 1860.

into a snake. The pharaoh asked his wise men and magicians, and the Egyptian magicians also started the ritual — each one threw his cane and it turned into a snake; but Aaron's cane devoured all others.

Remarks to magical and snake canes

To this day the voodoo cults in Haiti and Brazil use metal canes in snake form for their initiation rites, similar to the ones in Dahomey used by the Fon. The term Voodoo = Wodun = Magic originated in their language. In the middle ages magic canes in snake form did exist, but during that period there was a change in the meaning: the snake, the double symbol, which intrigues and disgusts us, became a symbol for earth and fertility. Besides this, the snake could be easily carved curving around the staff and became a common decoration. The snake cane can also be found as "Schulzenstab" worn as a symbol for law and order by the mayor of rural communities. (J.M. Ritz)

Magic

What do magic canes used by magicians in black satanic magic look like? Illustration 127 shows a cane from the collection of J.P. Favand: a devil's face is carved of human bones and the shaft is covered with human skin. The collection of G.J. Yorke holds the cane of the magician Aleister Crowley. It is wood, with a carved satan's head with flames coming out of it. Snakes are winding around the shaft, which bears the inscription "The Beast 666." This refers to the anti-christ from the book of Revelation, with whom Crowley identifies.

Magician canes can also look harmless. In magic books, such as Barrett's "The Magus," 1801, or in "Schluessel Salomons" they are illustrated and their making described: one has to cut at sun rise a twig from a hazel tree with a blood stained knife, cover it with pentagons and other magic symbols or one has to put special nails in it. Then it has to be sacrificed.

Or one could use a beggar's cane and convert it into a magic cane, because beggars often have the evil eye. "Krueitzens Ecyclopaedia" from Goethe's times sees it more simply, "a magic cane, a small cane, which is used by magicians, pocket player or charlatans to perform their acts or tricks by pointing at the object which would be changed while saying hocus pocus." There are system canes which are magic canes, holding scarfs, a second cane or even a small table.

The Roman Auguren carried crooked staffs with which they drew squares in the sand or pointed to the skies while giving their predictions. This so called lituus is the origin of the royal scepter — the byzantine Emperor Arcadius (395-408) carried such a short crook staff — and the bishop's staff. The most frequent explanation is that it has its origin in the shepherd's staff. The bishops were successors of Christ the good shepherd, fulfilling his demand to guard his flock.

Because the bishop's staff, until the concordance in Worms at the end of the "investiture argument," was given to the bishop by the Emperor during his inauguration, as a symbol of his vested power, as symbol of his authority of command and his power to judge, it was not considered part of his church ornat, but a worldly symbol. The third interpretation: it originated in the command staffs of the Roman empire. Either way, the baculus pastoralisit symbolizes the bishop's power, the church's power vested in him and the resulting spiritual power.

Initially they did not have any particular form; they were man high with a small cross or ball at the tip. They could be slightly curved like the crook of a chamois or had a t-form end. These types of crooks were usually made of ivory, and ended in animal heads curving slightly downward. A small hollow in the ivory crook would sometimes house relics. This type of crook disappeared during the 12th century in the Roman Catholic church, while it is still used in the orthodox churches today. However, the crooks are turned upwards and the symbol of a cross is in the middle of the staff.

The crook, which originally looked like the letter f, curved more and more until the circle closed. The closed circle was filled with symbolic figures. These could have been doves or lambs or unicorns. One of the latter, for example, is in Fulda, the material is ivory. While the romanic bishop's and abbot's shafts also had a snake and dragon biting the cross symbol, they were replaced by Mary and cross scenes. These were typically made of metal, silver or gilded bronze and a set with gem stones.

Staffs of priests, bishops and pilgrims

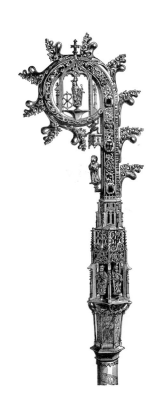

Fig. 5 Gothic crook from the Benedictine Monastery Saint Peter in Salzburg, 15th century.

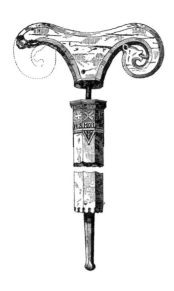

Fig. 6 Pastoral crook in early medieval form with silvered copper bands, Saint Peter, Salzburg

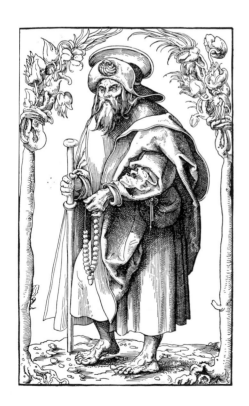

Fig. 7 Apostle Jacob as pilgrim; wood cut by Lukas Cranach the Older; circa 1510.

The symbolism of the bishop's staff is as follows: it should be pointed at the bottom, to sting the lazy and fight against sin; straight in the middle, to rule over the weak and to help the tumbling; crooked at the top, to collect the mistaken and pull them back. The bishop carried the staff with the crook pointing outward, since he ruled over everybody whereas the abbot carried the crook pointing over his shoulder because he only ruled the monastery.

Bishop's staffs are the symbols of Saint Nicholas and Saint Benno. Saint Kolomann carries a pilgrim's staff and Saint Wendelin a Shepherd's staff.

The lay priests in the Christian church of Ethiopia carried praying canes, which end in decorated iron or brass handles. They were used as aides during hours long ceremonies but also as symbols and rhythmic aides during singing and dancing.

The pilgrims' staffs were symbol, walking aide and weapon. We are familiar with them from many illustrations. As an example, on Hans Burgkmair's print "Pilger im Wald" (Pilgrim in the Forest): The shoulder high staff ends with a knob, after about 50 cm it has a symbolic ring. The staff is held between the ring and the knob or at hip height. Some staffs have hooks to hang food, which the pilgrim begged for. The pilgrim's position, many of whom walked across Europe in large numbers to reach the grave of Saint Jacob in Santiago de Compostela in North Western Spain, is unclear. Sometimes they were considered as annoying beggars, sometimes as devout people who received a special blessing for staff and bag by the church, the benedictio baculi et perae.

The medieval *wallestab* (in French "bourdon") of the pilgrims, originally was simple and functional, but later turned ornate, carved or painted, sometimes carrying an inlaid image of a saint and sometimes (as in Surpierre, Canton Fribourg, Switzerland, where the cane of Saint Magdalen is worshipped) the cane itself turns into a miraculous image. Max von Boehn describes several precious pilgrim staffs made of ivory, silver and gold decoration in his "Beierk der Mode." They had probably been used for pilgrim costumes which were quite popular at court. Pilgrims were also part of processions, which in Muehldorf/Inn were so frequent and popular at the beginning of the 19th century that they were referred to as "Steckenprozessionen" — cane processions.

The Pfarrerstoecke — priest's canes — were decorated with religious symbols (see illustrations 6 & 7), a special type of which was the Capuchin cane. Priest Wiebel, Kaufbeuren, describes it in 1937 as follows: "The Capuchine cane has a crooked handle, which is so narrow that it can not be worn over the sleeve, but hangs on the wrist on the naked skin, in order not to fall during reading or begging. My own cane was made in such a way that the crook similar to a head peeks from underneath the hood; below the handle the pictures of the founders of the begging orders, Saint Augustin for the Augustines, Franz von Assisi for the Franciscans and Capuchins, were applied."

The Marshal's baton is the most famous one, developed from the command batons. Originally rank signs of the Roman army, they appear in illustrations and portraits during the 16th century. The Marshal's batons are short, undecorated canes carried by the commander in his hands. It appears that the lower the rank, the more ornate the baton. Since the 18th century French Field Marshals carried the "baton fleurdelise," which was covered with blue velvet, with ornate needle point decoration and gilded ends. The Prussian generals carried command batons (30 cm long) covered with pale blue velvet, with applied gilded crowns and eagles and golden diamond covered rims, similar to the one Molke received for his 90th birthday. From 1900 onward admirals carried the admiral's baton, which had a secondary baton set with a telescope. While the baton itself was used during parades, the secondary one was carried on board. Four German grand admirals carried the imperial baton, two under Hitler. The last two were made by the jeweler Wilm in Berlin. They measured 49 cm long and had silver shafts covered with navy blue velvet, emblems (Reichs eagle, Iron cross and Anquor) in gold and a platinum submarine. The army field marshals also carried such batons.

English officers until the Second World War carried a swagger stick, a privately made symbol of their rank made of wood, horn or rhino with small crests or initials on silver knob.

The corporal's baton was a sign for lower officers. In Krunitz's encyclopedia it is described as follows: "a short Spanish cane (which was initially in several armies and in a few even now) worn by corporals and lower officers, and which was used during the exercising of new recruits. Frequently the corporal was ordered by the captain to punish a soldier with a certain number of strokes with the cane. All of this gave the cane the reputation of an exquisite means of punishment."

The canes of the secular powers

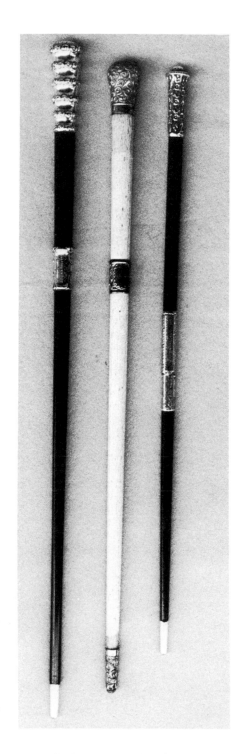

Fig. 8 Dedication canes, wood with silver mounts, whale bone, gild mounting. English, circa 1900.

Potsdam canes were made of lacquered wood, they looked similar to Spanish cane, and they were first offered by Sergeant Vietgow from the Kalkstein regiment. In 1764 the term was used all over Braunschweig and then all over Germany, in the nordic countries and also in America, according to the period writer Friedrich Nicolai. No special merit for the residence on the Havel? The traveling French man Risbeck wrote to his brother: "no army treats its recruits as soft as the Prussian one ... with respect to the cane, it is only used when the man is too stupid, clumsy, sloppy or malicious." The word from Austria is different "everywhere the almighty cane is ready." In October 1817 during the Wartburg gathering of students an Austrian corporal's cane, a Prussian military corset and a soldier's plait of hair were burned. This was the end of an era.

The "tambourmayors" of the French army and the Prussian drummers carried canes which had a gold or brass knob of silver, decorated with tassels and bands, which indicated the beginning and end of musical pieces. They are related to conductors' batons, which during the 17th century, according to travel reports, were excessively large among the French, the size of billiard sticks. They were used by the conductor to beat time. They were invented by the French composer Jean Baptiste Lully. He later died from such a baton: during the performance of a Te Deum on January 8, 1687 in Paris after Louis XIV recovered from a serious illness, he injured his foot with the metal tip of his baton and died of blood poisoning.

Around 1500, cantors had received batons, which were more symbols of dignity than conductor's aides. The conductor's baton of today was started in the 19th century. The first baton wielding conductors were Spontini, Spohr, Weber and Mendelssohn and they were heavily criticized for it. Batons can be collector's items in memory of famous conductors or small objects "de vertu." They were produced beautiful wood, ivory, horn or narwhal with silver or gold mounting and were given as presents or dedications.

The porter's and concierge staffs in large elegant houses and palaces were status symbols. When guests were expected, the lackeys stood with long brown lacquered canes with gold or gilded knobs "en galla" in front of the open door. Similar staffs were used by stewards to announce guests by stamping the staff and shouting the name — a scene used in every costume film.

The canes carried by the executive branch of the law were more like weapons. Originally a type of spear, an actual or imitation halberd altered on a long stick. It was called a mediator, which in reality meant the following: if somebody could not be convinced with arguments, words, or orders, he was beaten with the cane. In Frankfurt the night guards until the 19th century carried huge canes made of oak, which originally had lamps. Later these were replaced with quadrangular shaped heavy knobs bearing the seals of the town. These canes appeared to be terrible weapons, whereas they were used for a peaceful purpose. The night guard's cane was passed from one guard to next over the course of the night and could be seen as a forerunner to the control watch.

The medieval bailiffs and mercenaries, who together with the guilds were the recruits for the civilian army, kept law and order, and carried white canes (without bark) as symbols and instruments. At the end of the last century this white cane was shortened to a punching stick, which in England is the symbol and the only weapon of the constable. Punching sticks as symbols are metal and decorated; punching sticks as weapons are simple and handy. The custom of painting them with initials and crests was kept alive until the beginning of this century.

The *Stockmeister* — Cane master — executed punishments "on the skin," corporal punishments: "cane shillings" were hits to the bottom, thirty for a fine of one shilling. They were not considered humiliating and were not public. The public corporal punishment with canes and sticks performed by an executor was dishonoring. Often the condemned was literally beaten out of town. In England the corporal punishment was stopped in 1948, in Ireland in 1968 and in Germany in 1923.

The judge's staff and the ruler's scepter lost its connection to the walking cane a long time ago. Nevertheless it should be mentioned at this point, because of its symbolic value. According to the Lex Ribuaria, one had to take an oath upon a hazel twig (hasla). Illustrations of court procedures since the 13th century show the judge with a scepter. This staff was the sign of judicial power, which could be transferred to a replacement. The judge could only act as a judge if he had his staff in hand. He had to take it in his had at the beginning of the session and keep it in hand. This explains the breaking of the staff as an irrevocable condemnation. The earliest documented such trial was on April 8 1516 in Ingolstadt.

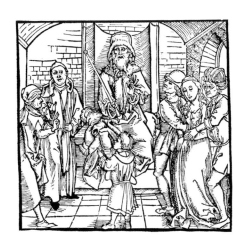

Fig. 9 The judge holds his cane upright, while Daniel presents his case in favor of Susannah. Woodcut by Albrecht Duerer (?), in "The Knight from Turn," Basel 1493.

Because the judges staff was the true symbol of the judge's power, it had to specially made. Wolfgang Schild writes the following in *Alte Gerichtsbarketi*, "A bad staff meant bad judging. Originally it should be without decoration, especially without bark under which demons could hide. The straight form is a remainder of old superstitions, the power of the world column or the pole as personification of ancestors. Only later, when these old superstitious and symbolic contents lost power and were forgotten, did the judges' staffs turn more and more to magnificent symbols of power and true court scepters." At some point they were replaced with the book of law.

The largest collection on judges staffs and scepters can be seen in the historical museum of Bern, Switzerland.

An extensive treatise has been written about academic scepters and staffs (which are sometimes still in use today) by Vorbrodt in 1971, containing many illustrations. Whether the royal scepter has its origin in the cane or the whip has not been researched. Charles the Great, besides his sceptrum consulare in the Frank's manner had a heavily decorated staff as an imperial emblem (baculus de arbore malo). His successor only used the scepter, mound, crown and sword as insignia.

From here on we will primarily focus on the walking stick.

The age of the walking and strolling cane

The philosophy behind the canes

Friedrich Nicolai, who from 1752 to 1811 ran the most famous book store in Berlin, wrote in his memoirs the following: "a walking cane is like the soft, unreal love, which, when difficulties arise does not withstand and which, instead of support, gives way. Just as nice and soft you appear, small vain thing, I can not praise you. A strong sturdy cane, cut from black thorn, on which I can lean, is much more to my liking." The canes Nicolai referred to may be seen in any number of fashion prints, they are more thin twigs than canes.

Johann Georg Kruenitz, the encyclopedic writer, sees it more objectively: "walking cane, a cane made of wood, bamboo, steel, fish bone etc., which is taken on walks either as a toy or as an actual walking aide. The toy canes are thin and flexible, the bamboo, steel or fish bone ones are strong and inflexible."

Walking, as a free and intentless encounter with nature, was discovered in the 18th century. At first in the planned gardens of the Tuileries, in Versailles and Fontainebleau, which had been designed by Andre Le Notre, and later in the century in the half wild parks of the English style. One promenaded, one chatted, flirted and underlined his nonchalance with a cane, which was rarely used to help with the walking. The cane represented and fortified the carrier's personality with a minimum of effort, compared to today's status symbol, the car. The cane was, in poets words, the exclamation mark of the inner and outer being.

How important the cane was for people in the landscape is confirmed by an article in *Antiquitaeten Zeitung* about a suite of porcelain from Wurzburg, made in the short period between the late fall of 1775 and the early summer 1780. The author is Dieter Schneider-Henn who wrote: "Never through the landscape without a cane." On every single piece of Wuerzburg porcelain he found a figure in the landscape: a man with a cane, and a woman with a cane on the chocolate pot. "Once this detail is discovered, one focuses on the detail of how the cane is worn. It seems that the cavaliers of the 18th century were well versed in handling the cane. It was used as support, elegantly under the arm, over the shoulder or they carried it as a pointer in front. Whether standing or sitting they always have the cane in hand, and if two figures were grouped, the painter equipped them sometimes both with cane."

At the time a cane was an integral part of the life of a certain social class. It was considered a symbol of culture and nobility

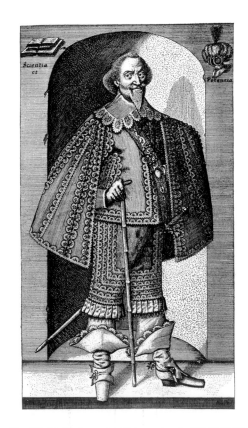

Fig. 10 *Duke August of Braunschweig (1568-1636) wearing the typical long, oversized cane. Copper etching by an unknown artist.*

(which later had nothing to do with birth). It was not considered useful as a walking aide, just as there are beautiful but not necessarily useful things with which we surround ourselves.

The Alamode cavalier

The Spanish cavalier, because of the superior power of the Spanish court, was the example for all of Europe. He almost always carried a sword, which showed his rank. The sword was highly decorated with chasing and gold and silver inlay. The cane as a male accessory did not exist yet. With the disappearance of the Spanish costume — the pendulum of taste suddenly moving from the noble austere to the sloppy plain — the cane suddenly appeared. The cavalier Alamode (in the latest fashion) from 1630 on carries, in addition to his sword and plate size spurs, a straight cane with a knob and, sometimes, a decorative band. In the "Alamodischen Discurs" (high fashion conversation) between a dandy and his Famulus (private secretary) on a pamphlet of the period the most interesting section for our purpose reads: "Dandy. 25 What else can one say about the cane and commander / which we tend to carry / always in hand / ? - Famulus. 26 One says, if one takes away everything from the dandy, he is still left with his cane to guard off the dogs." In the corresponding prints they are casually leaning against their canes, which usually have strong iron tips. Even if this fashion only lasted until the second half of the 17th century, the cane became a fashion requisite for the next 300 years. The first King permanently wearing a cane was Louis XIII. It was a straight cane made of spotted wood of same diameter from top to bottom. In the copper prints of Abraham de Bose, which narrate the daily life of Louis XIII, he never misses his cane. At the reception for the Parisian merchants in 1628, the cane could have been crowned with an ivory apple, which the newspaper "L'Art du dix-neuvieme siecle" mentioned.

Canes certainly existed before which were neither walking aides nor power symbols. But those were the exceptions, such as in the inventory of Henry VIII's palace in Greenwich or on a portrait of Sir G. Hart in Lullingstone, Kent from 1587. The cane shafts had highly ornate upper sections, they were grabbed right under the knob, made of chase metal and had metal tips to give hold in the ground. Other royal canes are described by Max von Boehn in his earlier discussed book. Among the ivory canes shown in

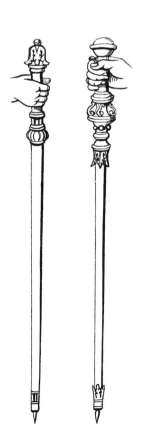

Fig. 11 Canes from the 16th century: the one on the left illustrated in a memorial plate in the cathedral of Salisbury (1578); the one on the right from a portrait of Sir G. Hart, 1587, in Lullingstone/Kent

Boehn's book is illustration 297 of Duke Albrecht V of Bavaria and his cane with a golden sun dial as a knob. A sabarcane, a weapon for killing birds, had been transferred into a little cane for Maria de Medici, on behalf of the ruler Louis XIII. Through the hollow blowing cane, the lady's were blown candy, wrapped in paper printed with proverbs. Because this fun could also hit the eye, it eventually was forbidden. And during Louis' time, these were replaced with the walking cane.

Change of fashion

The slouch hatted Alamode cavalier was followed by the round hatted dandy, whose social manners were full of theatrical mannerisms. He always had a medium strong cane in his right hand, which he played with when walking down the road. English authors like Ben Jonson called it "Straddling" (walking with legs wide apart). During the Queen Anne period, at the turn of the new century, the gallant followed, always wearing a muff, because his lower arms were only shirt covered, and a cane on a band and bow. In a poem, describing the market on the frozen Themse in 1684 it says: "a spark of the bar with his cane and his muff." During the Rococo, when the allonge headpiece was replaced by the pony tail, the cane is so important, that it is illustrated on an allegorical copper print about fashion as the only accessory. Three different styles are shown, the knob, the bec de corbin and the Fritz handle. The first young people are seen wearing only a cane, leaving out the sword. In England the sword had already disappeared from public life and was only used during ceremonies. In 1772 a group of young people imported some Italian fashions after a trip to Italy and, contrary to the arch conservative beef-steak club, started the macaroni club. The macaronis had a very high combed hair style crowned by a small hat. The hat was raised with a cane. The cane was very long and decorated with wide silk scarves which had found their opposite in wide silk neck scarves. The French revolution put an end to this courtly fashion, which was carried on by servants and lackeys — the black jacket became the festive outfit of the bougoise. In June 1790 a fashion statement from Paris said: "The wheel of fashion is very sturdy. We continue to dress ourselves English."

In 1786 F.J. Bertuch and G.M. Kraus published the first German fashion magazine called "Journal des Luxus und der Moden."

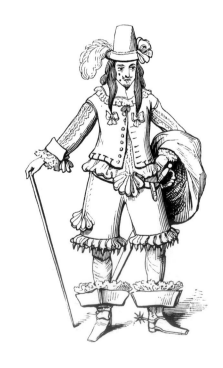

Fig. 12 An English dandy, wearing a round hat, around 1645, who, because of the boots, had to walk bow legged.

The following are articles from the first 17 editions, the later ones did not mention canes:

Paris, September 1, 1786: The good tone requires ladies to wear a long cane on the morning promenade, in the afternoon a light badine or a bamboo. The classification was: Cannes, bambous, wangees, toncs, racines and vignes. These are the cane categories according to etiquette. If one is bon-ton, one has to win them all. In Paris there are stores specializing in the sale of canes.

(Badine is a thin whip; cannes are lone canes; bambou = bamboo; wangee=pearl bamboo; tonc=peppercane; racines=root canes; vignes=vines)

Vienna, May 14, 1788: The gentlemen's cane is a thin bamboo, which has a thin gold plate instead of the knob!

Paris, January 6, 1792: The gentlemen's winter outfit includes a large sword cane.

Latest fashion from Germany, March 10, 1792: They still carry the knot cane (the English), most usually shouldered like a gun.

London, September 24, 1792: ... a short thorn cane, thick at the base and pointed at the top, for defense, in hand (the illustrated cane is about 50 cm long)

Berlin, May 8, 1793: The male puppet has a rhinoceros cane in hand and is filled with about 1 to 2 pounds of lead; here you have our current Hercules Adonisse and lowering hope of the states ... The portrait of the unhappy murdered King Louis XIV is on every piece of decoration and fashion; the most beautiful and exceptional invention was a small tuned cane knob made of ebony, the parts of which add up to the most realist silhouette of the kings head, if the cane is held away form the eye against a white wall. Speculation is, that it is an invention of French royalists, which wear these knobs on their canes as a sign of mourning.

From Germany, March 10 1796 ... and an American cane made of hickory tree. (in reference to the English influence on German fashion).

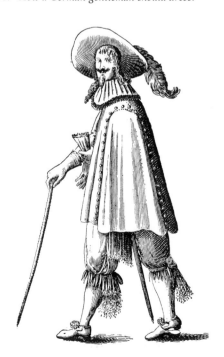

Fig. 13 The Alamode cavalier as seen on a pamphlet in 1630: "How a German gentleman should dress."

Hamburg, November 1799: The walking bats and sticks (practical expression of human rights, as they were called by one writer) become rarer and rarer and are replaced by small canes which at top and bottom are applied with silver, which by nature do not reach the ground, and can be used to occupy the hands.

Hamburg, February 19, 1802: Our young gentlemen now carry peace canes, which are little sticks, used to make peace and keep peace.

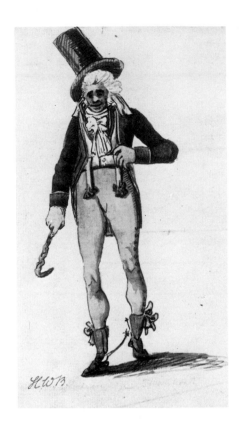

Fig. 14 *The cavalier with three vests and the knotted cane. Water color by H.W. Bunburry, circa 1805.*

It is interesting to note at this point, that the cane changed permanently, even more than fashion. There were also cane forms such as clubs or switches, which were not kept or collected as canes. If they ever had handles worth saving they were probably mounted on a straight, normal shaft. When looking at fashion prints from as late as the middle of the 19th century, one sees little more than regular canes. I do not believe that there are only stylistic and artistic reasons behind it. I assume that many of the small handle which have been saved and are mounted on long, thin shafts and are called lady's canes originally had been handles on short gentlemen's canes. Amazing also, that one rarely sees the image of one of those figural knobs, which are offered in large numbers today. Also, at the end of the 19th century most illustrated canes were simple knobs, straight handles and crooks handles.

The knot cane, the cork screw cane of the Jacobins, was adapted by the incroyables (= the unbelievables), which were the strange "jeunesse dore" (= gilded youth or young people of wealth and fashion) of the French republic. Usually sons of parvenu, they roamed the streets and restaurants, which Max von Boehn wrongly interpreted as brave opposition against the Jacobins. Together with their girls, the merveilleuses (the marvelous ones), the punks of their time, all wore long, neglected hair styles en oreilles de chien (like dog's ears), and custom made but intentionally ill fitting tail coats unevenly buttoned. The secret salute was a rhythmic lifting and lowering of the cane.

When the dandies came in around 1812, regular canes were worn again and the knot cane was "roroco," which was the term for anything out of fashion. In the 1830s, dandies became swells, who replaced the dandy's tie with a glove craze. At about this time Honore de Balzac started his cane cult. According to Baron von Eelking: "The talk around Balsac's canes was instrumental in the cane's position in fashion for many decades, not least of which were valuable specimens of elegant top hat canes." The last reference was probably made because Eelking's book "The image of the elegant man" is a guide to top hats. During the 1850s, long ivory handles were developed, which had either a straight handle, or a pistol handle form and were carved with armorial crests, emblems of fraternities, or hunting scenes. They were mainly made in the Dresden or Schlesia region.

The golden age of canes was between 1830 and the beginning of the First World War. It was not only part of fashion and outfit, but part of the personality. One carried the cane which fit the occasion and mood. One displayed it with images on the handles of the fierce teeth of a boxer, the smile of a Chinese, the muscular elegance of a horse or the symbol of an empty skull. Around 1890 the Quarter around Rue Saint-Denis, Saint-Martin and Saint-Sauveur had over 250 shops specializing in canes. Slowly the more elegant ones moved to better quarters. A similar development took place in London and canes could cost a fortune.

This was the time of artistically decorated handles and of system canes. System canes were either hiding something, had several functions, or were simply created as gags.

Canes also became important in the United States of America, according to a report in the "Leipziger Illustrierte" of August 25, 1883: "In America currently the cane is the most cherished fashion article for men — supposedly because it helps prevent the bad habit of the American of putting his hands in his pockets, which one tries to stop. This article therefore receives much more attention there than here. The dandies of the New World have their own fashion magazines dedicated to canes, just as ladies had their luxury article magazines, and the true swell chooses his cane with much thought and attention. First it was the whale bone cane, then the latest fashion asked for tiny, crooked canes similar to shepherd's canes, followed by the curved cane made of wood, which was referred to as "zulu" and which was imported from Paris. Last year the cane with silver knob was ahead of his brothers; the shaft had to be made of some rare wood; either the Chinese whonga because of its regular knotting or orande and lemon tree wood or myrthe, ebony, cactus or rose wood, the most popular is the wood of a palm tree growing on the island of Malacca.

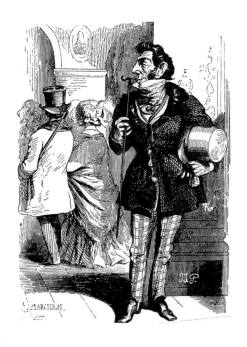

Fig. 15 "The Parisian Dandy," woodcut by Grandville for 1841 in the magazine "Le Prisme."

The manufacture ... is mainly done in New York, and the cane industry feeds many families there." (with respect to the fashion statements this article is just as unreliable a source as such articles usually are).

The last fashionable canes were thick Manila canes around 1927. But they do not have the same flair.

When the cane turned into a fashion accessory for the man of world, ladies did not want to stand aside and leave the cane to men. There are three reasons women wanted canes, which occurred in chronological order. First there was emancipation: the cane was treasured as much by women as by men, second there were practical reasons to carry a cane in times of high heels, and thirdly it was the joy as a playful fashion accessory.

The first intentional female cane carriers were the feminine opponents of Cardinal Mazarin. The rebel ladies, lead by the Duchess of Montpensier, carried canes to demonstrate their good and rebellious intentions. The cane of the Duchesse is documented: it was short, the knob was decorated with ribbons in the colors of the fronde. In 1649 it was used to start the cannons on the Bastille to fire against the royal troops.

At the same time, court costume including a cane was worn on theater stages. The actresses wore very high heels which made them taller than the men on stage, and used canes to walk on stage. These canes were lacquered and had a knob on which to lean.

Ladies, who about 100 years earlier had used the Venetian zoccoli, were supported by two servants when they walked on their 20 cm thick soles. Around 1751, when heels once again grew longer, they used canes, as is described in the "women's lexicon" of Amaranthes : "on several places they use canes decorated with ribbons for walking." Queen Sophie Charlotte went supported by a cane, inlaid with her monogram in gild wire and metal stones, on her walks with Leibniz. Another 50 years later, ladies again wore high heels but chose to be carried in sedan chairs. The very high coiffures were supported by sticks, which were carried by servants, according to period prints.

The cane had a small bottle in its handle containing smelling salts, a powder compartment, and a folding fan. Sometimes these

Lady's canes

Fig. 16 "La promenade du matin," copper etching after Sigmund Freudenberger, etching from 1774.

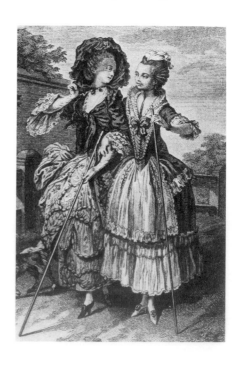

canes were combined with umbrellas, which were set under the handle. The disadvantage of this arrangement was that if one wanted to use the umbrella, one had to hold the part of the cane in hand which usually touched the ground.

When the fashion changed for ladies toward a more male dress code with the redingote (= gentlemen's coat which is fitted to the waist), the badine (= rod) in hand was more important. Fifty years later, around the middle of the century, ladies started smoking in public and, of course, also wore a walking stick. By 1890, some felt it was difficult to distinguish men from women on the street.

At the end of the last century, J. Charlemont was quite upset about: "the bathers form Trouville, the female tourists, the lady's of the world, who came to the Spa or who strolled in Vichy, had a cane in hand and acted in a masculine way, which in the eyes of respectable men was unsuitable for married women or mothers." The author rejected the lady's cane "because one leans on a cane which is not necessary for women, thanks to their natural harmonic composure. Man carry canes because otherwise he would not know what to do with his hands, and it allows him, like a cigar in his mouth, to make certain gestures, which hide his nervousness. Ladies are charming by nature."

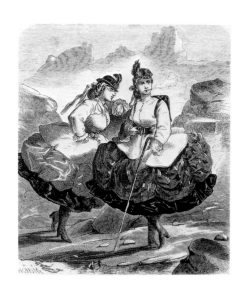

Fig. 17 The travel costume in the mountains: fashion cartoon by Herbert Koenig form 1867 in "Gartenlaube."

The use of the cane

Even if the cane is used in a language of gestures to hide nervousness, it is a language which has to be learned. A little book about how to prevent accidents with canes and umbrellas provided helpful tips. In 1808 the second edition of this book was printed, "Hints to the Bearer of Walking Sticks and Umbrellas." The author used the assumed name "Solomon Supplejack." Before citing from this amusing and important book for the cane industry, I would like to add a few personal notes.

First you should take a walking stick and walk with it. It is not easy, especially if you want to appear elegant. The rhythm of tapping-the-ground and raising high-in-the-air has to be just right. Because the walking stick should be part of your appearance, it should not be used to hide or assist a hobbling and limping gait. Try to handle a cane, preferably in front of a mirror. There are many people who are naturals (which was much more important in earlier times), but most of us have to simply learn it. I have been in training for two years to casually use a cane and I am making some progress. I take a cane on all my walks. It pleases the palm, sometimes acts as a pillar, loosens my steps and — even if it sounds sentimental — it is a good companion. However, I live in the countryside. A cane is not as nice in town. I never use one in a social setting. Our Mr. Supplejack talks the great nuisance walking stick bearers are to their fellow pedestrians.

At the beginning of the last century, the sidewalks were very narrow and canes were very frequent. This should explain some of the complaints voiced: "The sidewalk is a public place, but there has to be some limit to ones use of it. If one person, without any consideration for the comfort of others, uses the room of 4 to 6 people, one in all fairness has to call him a public nuisance and one has to try to stop this behavior." This public nuisance is, of course, the walking stick bearer. For example: "A gentlemen unintentionally puts his walking stick in the mud of the road and, without any bad intentions, rather thoughtlessly wipes the cane clean on the passing lady's clean dress. Another gentleman swirls his cane in the air, well knowing that eventually it will hit someone, break a lamp, or will catapult the street mud on the back and in the faces on people in front or in the back. A third gentleman holds his cane tight under his arm. He might poke a pedestrian who is following him in a faster pace in his eye, or, should the carrier bend over, hits the following pedestrians body or soils his cloth. If he turns around, he turns into a turnstile: his cane rules the whole sidewalk. The passing pedestrians are his in the back and in the face and everybody is forced to make way. The biggest damage is done by those who use their cane in an outward direction, in order to make more room for themselves and everybody who is not paying attention to their steps inevitably will take a fall."

The conclusion to avoid any of these situations: "The walking stick and the umbrella have to be carried as close to the body as possible, upright and on the front. I refrain from telling young gentlemen, that nothing is graceful, which is contrary to usefulness."

Rules about the proper use of the walking stick can be found in magazines and fashion books. According to the "Tatler" magazine a gentleman named Isaak Biekerstaff had founded an academy in 1710 (the article did not mention where it had been founded), which taught the proper use of the cane and smelling salts. I could not find any confirmation that an academy for gracious and gentle use of the walking stick had ever been founded as suggested by the author.

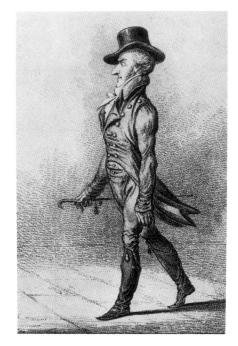

Fig. 18-21 How to wear ones cane in London around 1800. Fashion character studies, prints

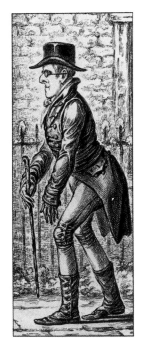

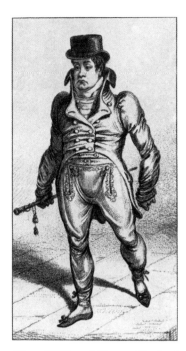

by James Gilray (1802) and Thomas Rowland (1789).

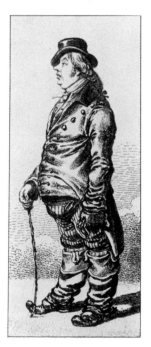

The same article says "I love my cane like a third leg. How could I ever lead a smart conversation or be seen in society without, from time to time, poking my cane at my shoe, resting my leg on it or how could I whistle?" The publishers Steel and Addison certainly wanted to ridicule the fashion of the decorative cane.

In all, the know-how of wearing a cane is hard to learn from theoretical descriptions. It has to be acquired through daily practice. There were people who refused to follow the trend. Jacob Grimm writes to Achim von Arnim in 1822: "I can not get myself to take a cane and to walk down the road with dignity." But, the walking stick was worth thinking and writing about.

Much can be learned about the use of walking sticks by studying period prints and cartoons. It was improper to carry the cane in ones coat pocket, yet it was done during the Biedermeier period. Otherwise it is carried under the arm, the hand around the knob, which pushed the cane slightly upwards. Or one carries it in both hands like a procession candle, one rests it in the shoulder or turns it between the fingers. One other odd way of carrying the cane: one holds the cane by the lower third of the shaft, the handle upside down. This was the way to carry the cane in the first quarter of the twentieth century. This was fashionable and had a practical purpose: If the handle is too heavy and the cane is top-heavy, the handle tilts to the back when the cane is held only loosely at the shaft.

The ideal cane is lightweight, made of Malacca cane, with the equilibrium about two hand widths below the handle: it is always well balanced, not matter how it is carried. How canes were carried in the Belle Epoche is best discussed by Baron von Eelking, the cane expert for that period. Only canes with straight handle, almost exclusively made of ivory, were actual walking aides and did beat the walking rhythm on the pavement. Canes with crooked handles were hung on the arm or held in hand in order to have something in hand. The tail coat cane (usually made of black or blackened woods, with gold mountings and an ivory ball, a cabochon cat eye or rock crystal knob) was worn to the opera. It was squeezed under the left arm while promenading during intermission, but it was not used as a walking stick. One might possibly lean on it casually or used it to wave a coach or cab.

The tail coat cane survived as an important requisite of the tap dance for 30 years longer than the walking stick.

Many of the subjects discussed so far were only valid for people of rank: to carry a cane was considered a privilege. In Brandenburg, around 1600, only peasants fiefed by the Elector were allowed to carry carved and ribboned canes. Everybody else was punished with a labor camp for up to one year for carrying a cane. Whoever wore a cane in the presence of the Czar in Russia was beheaded. Catherine the Great made use of this law on her cross country and hunting visits, if peasants or civilians did not throw their cane away fast enough when bowing their head while the Empress passed by.

Theoretically the Insignia laws of the Magna Charta are still valid in England. Judges could still punish a civilian for carrying a cane in a closed room or carrying a gold decorated cane. During the French Revolution the carrying of canes was permitted. A law which was revoked by Napoleon in 1804. Informant Charlemont saw it as follows: "In France the cane is prohibited from entering theaters, museums and other public places, a mistake which one does not know how to change. If the civilian is forced to leave his cane in the wardrobe, why not also force the soldiers to leave their swords and daggers; those are much more dangerous weapons than our simple and weak walking sticks. On the stormy evening of the performance of 'Germanicus' on March 22, 1812, which later was referred to as the Bataille des Cannes (= Battle of the Canes), all sorts of canes (joncs, bambous et rotins) were lifted for and against the authors, one also saw some swords. After that more and more people started wearing swords to places where canes had been prohibited."

After the July Revolution in 1830, Louis Philippe of Orleans became the successor of his cousin Charles X. Because Charles had always worn a gold decorated cane in public, Louis Philippe started wearing an umbrella. During his reign, which was marked by civil unrest, Grandville published a lithograph "the nightmare of the chief of police or the mutiny of walking sticks and umbrellas," which as printed in "La Caricature" on July 21, 1831 and which made fun of the cane prohibition (three years later swords were also prohibited) and which showed the cane as a potential weapon. When, after the unrest of the laborers, the followers of Charles started a conspiracy against "the Pear" (La Poire was the nickname for the King and he wear referred to as Pear), Louis Philippe was suddenly seen with a knob cane: the peaceful umbrella days were passed. This almost lead to another unrest. The

General cane prohibitions

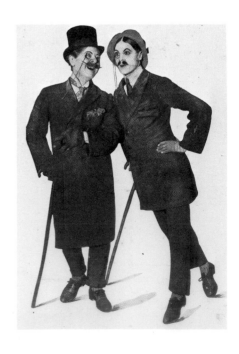

Fig. 22 The Music Hall comedians Ike and Will Scott with their Tap canes, around 1920.

Fig. 23 "The mutiny of the canes and umbrellas," litho-graph by Cranville, 1831.

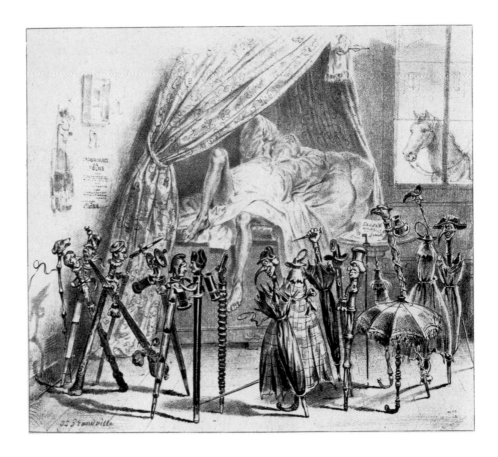

revolution followed in 1848. It started in Paris, continued in Berlin and was quite bloody in March. One of the demands of the revolutionaries was the lifting of many useless rules. One of those rules was the one governing the prohibition of canes for certain segments of the population, which King Friedrich Wilhelm IV lifted on August 16. During the course of one month over 1 million canes were sold in Berlin.

While earlier portraitists paid little attention to the design of the cane handle, there are many designers' drawings and, after 1850, also catalogues which allow the proper identification and dating of cane handles. Metal canes can be dated if they are hall-marked for date or bear a maker's mark, if they bear an inscription referring to somebody known, or even a date; however, any kind of inscription could have been added at a later date, whenever the cane changed owner. With engravings, a cane could also be made to appear older, or with a dedication to a famous person be made more valuable. If the cane has a carved handle, whatever the material, the question of provenance and age is almost impossible to answer. Also style-wise many questions can not be answered. "Is the bust Renaissance or Neo-renaissance? When was this cane carved, during the 18th, 19th or 20th century?" Collectors and dealers have the tendency to make canes older, and an engraving or a date is gratefully believed to be correct, even if it is an unlikely 16th century date.

During the 17th and 18th century most canes had knobs. In England, the knob was generally made of ivory or rhinoceros horn, with applied silver nails, referred to a "pique."

On the continent, depending on the means of the owner, cane knobs were made of gold, silver, or gilded or silvered metal. In 1733, the Crown prince of Bayreuth received from his father-in-law, the Soldier King Friedrich Wilhelm I, a cane knob made of Princemetal (= a non-tarnishing brass alloy), since the King hated luxury. He had on his own canes gilded glass knobs, which Queen Sophie Dorothee purchased at the Potsdam glass works for the standard price of 1 taler per piece. Knobs made of porcelain were also quite economical, they were offered between 1 and 60 Dukaten by the newly founded porcelain manufactories and were usually offered in three styles: the knob form, the Bec de Corbin (ravens peak — which was only slightly curved), and the T-form handle, also called (after its most famous bearer) the "Fritz handle." The greek letter Tau, which is slightly upwards and downwards curved at the end, is the best name for the most popular German cane handle.

A collection of beautiful French gold knobs from pre-revolutionary times can be seen at the Musee des Arts Decoratifs in Paris. Another noteworthy collection was the Rothschild collection, which was auctioned in May 1975 by Sotheby's in Monaco. Illustration 13 shows a handle with a combination of gold and enamel.

Handles and their dating

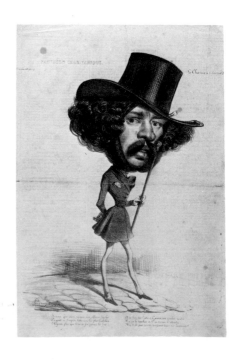

Fig. 24 The artist Paul Gavarni is shown with fashionable top hat and cane in the Parisian magazine "Charavarie," for which he also worked. Circa 1850.

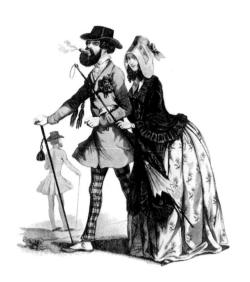

Fig. 25 "Frenzies and the latest fashions," the lady's with her mother's hat and her great great aunt's cane; the gentleman with tassel cane, Scottish pants and Irish hat. Satirical print from "Wiener Theaterzeitung," circa 1850.

Most of the canes were made of tri-color gold, with chased figures, garlands and acanthus leaf decoration. They were originally owned by important leaseholders or tax collectors, by professionals whose professions allowed the carrying of canes (which were sign of a class, as will be discussed later), and by doctor's. Other materials used during this period were amber, tortoise, gold set or decorated with gem stones like jaspis or turquoise, and set with diamonds. The shaft was malacca cane and long enough to be held just below the handle to fully display its decoration. For special occasions canes were made of cloudy agate, kept in fitted leather cases. Lord Petre in Alexander Popes "Lockenraub" (The thief of the lock) owns such a cloud cane. More economical, decorative alternatives were the painted, long canes from the Louis XVI period (see illustration 11).

Because of the rather dirty roads, until the 19th century canes had a long brass ferrule, with or without a pointed tip or an attached iron pin. They did not exist on courtly canes, but otherwise are a good time mark.

Figural handles were rare until the 19th century. Ivory handles were made as animals, figures and heads, often carved by the same carvers, who worked on silver ware handles and often a silverware handle would end up as a cane handle. The Tau handles, which ended in turkish heads, pugs and ladies busts were also figural. Other examples are porcelain ladies with or without veils. The Georgian cavaliers carried canes as described in the "London Chronicle" of 1762 which had knobs covered with waxed threads or ivory knobs the size of silver pennies. The elaborate figural knobs were popular after 1830. In 1899 we can read in J. Charlemont's historical notes about the cane "which is taken on walks, decorated and well formed. The simple civilian has it with a gilded apple, the dandy has it gem stone covered, the rioter has it with a sword, the old man with a girls head, the fashion addict with a silver ring, the retiree with a black horn, the show-off with a lead end to defend himself against anybody who ridicules him." From the Biedermeier period on, canes were manufactured industrially, which brought new techniques and specialists, making curved handles and crooks possible.

The cane as art object and social passport

Who made handles

Most canes were made anonymously, their history and maker unknown. Only a very few handle carvers and gold smiths are known by name: rarely did anybody sign their work; porcelain handles do not bear marks. Canes made of precious metals do have hallmarks which allow the dating of the cane, makers' marks are, unless by a famous maker, usually hard to identify. If the mark is in the ring, which is the setting between handle and shaft, it might be misleading because the handle could have been replaced.

Valid attribution is only possible with signed canes, stylistically unquestionable examples like the ones from the studio of Fabergé, some porcelain knobs or the industrially made canes, which are listed in catalogues. One can also recognize certain "hand writings" of carved ivory, or rare woods, where certain motifs reappear with small alterations.

By now I have come across three canes with boxers (see illustration 193), one is stained in two colors, the other one slightly longer and slimmer, due to the shape of the ivory. The artist was so well trained in carving this dog (a very popular breed at the time), that he carved it many times. If one looks at a large number of canes, one realizes that certain motifs are quite frequent and that certain models of a motif have been made several times. I am referring to custom-made canes and not industrially made canes, the handles of which were carved in specialized carving companies as piece work (of the over 100 handle manufactures in Germany 17 were specialized in ivory carving). Custom-made refers to the handle and shaft. However, the borders are unclear. A cane with a porcelain handle by Kaendler is certainly a custom-made cane, yet it was made by using a mold, which had been in use for 150 years. The figural pear wood handles of a carver in Thueringen seem to be unique, yet we know from a catalogue that they are carved in series. Now, let us try to list names.

Franz Anton Bustelli designed numerous porcelain cane handles, three of which are still made into bottle corks by the Nympehnburg Porcelain Manufacture. Bustelli also did some ivory carvings around 1740. Cane handles do exist by Joseph Teutschmann in Passau, the cane shown in illustration 6, 7 is from his circle. Johann Christoh Ludwid Lucke is also a known ivory carver who worked in Meissen and whose Form number 269, a male head with a silly cap has been used as a cane knob. This motif has surfaced as a porcelain knob many times. Johann Kaendler designed several porcelain handles. The handles with ladies heads are specifically mentioned in his work papers. Notes from January 1740: "1 cane handle with lady's head was inventoried and made in a rough form, to be further treated from inventory." This popular handle style was frequently copied by smaller manufactories.

A number of cane suppliers and jewelers, which delivered canes to the cane lover Friedrich II, are listed by Max von Boehn: "The merchant Gotzkaowskij delivered a cane handle made of mother of pearl, set in gold, for 125 Taler. The court jeweler Jordan delivered a gold knob for 35 Taler; a Bec de Corbin made of jasper, set in gold and applied with diamonds for 360 Taler; a circular enamel knob covered with diamonds for 2270 Taler and a four color gold cane for 1400 Taler." One should keep in mind though, that valuable canes, just as valuable porcelains, were considered capital investments and could be sold again. For example, the Soldier King did sell all of his father's, Friedirch I's diamond set canes.

Fig. 26 Catalogue entry with animal head handles made of pear tree, F. Jennert, circa 1900.

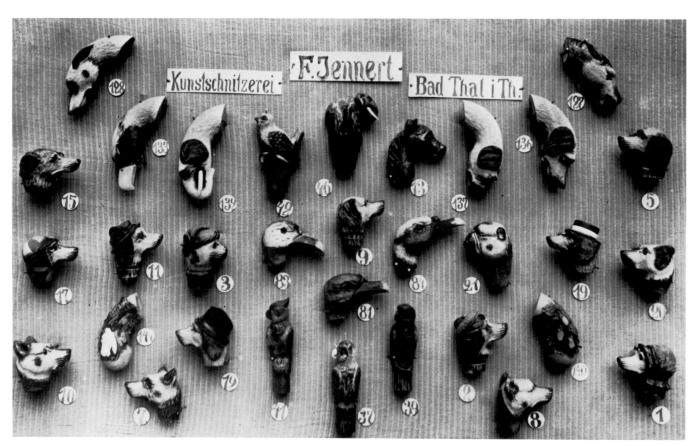

Pattern sheets list the names of jewelers Maria, Paris 1760 and Lalonde, Paris 1780. The previously mentioned Rothschild collection identifies Michel-Rene Bocher 1760-1791, Germian Chaye 1755-1788, Edme-Pierre Balzac 1739-1752 and Jean Ecosse 1705-1743. The same collection also included a cane by the Dresden court jeweler Johann Christian Neuber (1735-1765), who was a master in the pietra dura technique.

One has to assume, that most jewelers also made canes, but where are they now?

I would also like to name the artist Samuel Alba from Vienna, who is a good example for a 19th century cane maker. He received a special mention from the judges at the German Industrial Fair in Munich 1854 for an assortment of walking canes, usually bamboo, the artistically carved knobs of which have to be seen as works of art, and indeed are more useful as such than for their intended purpose, because the delicate carvings make a real use almost impossible, without danger of breaking the cane. Alba also has to be credited with beautiful carvings in meerschaum. It is also useful to this craft to compare styles.

A superior carving is found on canes by Deyhle in Markgroeningen in Wuerttemberg. While artistically not at all behind those previously mentioned, his canes did have a practical advantage, because the carving was set in away that it would not diminish the use of the knob. Such functional cane handles had also been designed by the director of the arts and crafts academy in Munich, Hermann Dyck, which were illustrated in the German Trade Magazine in 1891.

Carl Fabergé, who came to fame in 1884 when his first Easter egg was delivered to the Czar's family, was a gold smith by trade, but rarely did any work himself. He was the designer, the intuition and organizer. At times, he employed as many as 700 gold smiths, carver and enamel workers in his atelier in Petersburg. The following head masters are important: Erik Kolin until 1866; Michael Perchin until 1903; Henrik Wigstroem until the atelier was closed in 1918. The stone cutters worked anonymously.

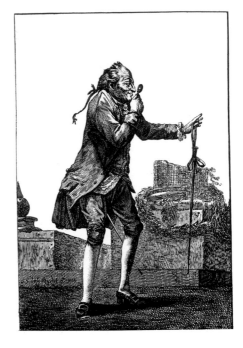

Fig. 27 *"Oh, look at the short skirt" portrait of a ladies man with decorative sword and cane by Joseph Franz von Goerz, circa 1780.*

Fabergé's specialties included: translucent enamel over engine turned gold in blue, orange and grey. The beauty of his enamel work has not been repeated since. One hundred forty four enamel

The canes by Carl Fabergé and his artisans

colors do exist, which in different layers can be either translucent or opaque in such a multitude of colors that each color seems unique. In order to achieve a brighter enamel shine, the silver round was covered with platinum. The carved stone objects, ranging from classic to trashy, are made of rock crystal, nephrit, serpentine, agate, lapislazuli, and obsidian, to name but the most common ones. Purpurin, a red glass material, was exclusively used by Fabergé. By the way, not everything that looks like it at first and second glance is indeed by Fabergé. Russian competition was already imitating his style during his life time, and Fabergé continues to be forged. The best characteristic of an original Fabergé is its exquisite quality. Between 1954 and 1980 the price for Fabergé objects has increased ten fold.

Among the famous artists of the Art Nouveau period, Rene Lalique made some beautiful figural silver handles and glass handles. Silver knobs were also designed by George de Feure, Rupert Carabin and "in the taste" of Alphonse Mucha.

A few good addresses for fine canes

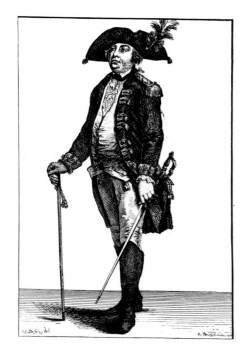

Fig. 28 "The Captain of the Guard" with sword and cane. Copper etching by Franz von Goerz, circa 1780.

In the nineteenth century, Thomas Briggs of London was one of the firms which signed the canes they sold. The handles were not manufactured by Briggs, but purchased from exclusive makers and jewelers and retailed by Briggs. The golden duck (illustration 203) is also signed CC for Charles Cooke, who actually made the object at the turn of the twentieth century. Cooke made many cane and whip handles in his jeweler's shop.

Briggs still exists: Swaine Adeney Briggs continues to sell umbrellas, canes, whips and fine leather goods. Another good London address is James Smith and Sons, Umbrella and Walking Stick Manufactures. On June 1893, James Smith, the "king of walking-stick manufactures" was quoted in "Answers" to the subject "some valuable walking sticks": "80 pounds for an unmounted malacca shaft — oh yes, this is quite possible — real, good Malacca cane is very valuable." Shortly before that the reporter had spotted in a window on the Boulevard Saint Germain in Paris a Malacca cane about five feet long for 2,000 Francs. Mister Smith thought the price was fair, such a cane, with even thickness, is unique, any shaft more than three feet long is very rare." "Also real snake wood — the most imitated wood — is very expensive. Ten pounds for a well marked shaft is the going price. The most expensive canes are made of rhinoceros horn. Rarely are the horns long enough to carve a shaft from them. Usually they are used for whips. A three feet four inch shaft always costs over 20 pounds, the horn only, without any mounting ... as a comparison, a thin whangee (pearl bamboo) can be purchased for nine shillings. The thicker it is, the more regular the knots, the more valuable. But never over 3 or 4 pounds ... a cane becomes much more expensive by its mounting. If gold and small gem stones are used, one should calculate 40 to 50 pounds. A perfect lady's cane, made of rhinoceros horn with a suitable gold handle will cost approximately 70 pounds, about the same as the best, thin Malacca cane. But the handle can make a cane much more expensive."

The leading cane stores in Paris were Antoine — in the arcades of the Palais Royal — Renard on the Place Victor Hugo, Bataille in the Rue Royale and Cazal on the Boulevard des Italiens. According to an article in the magazine "Sports" prices were around 750 Francs, with some as high as 2,000 - 3,000 Francs. And the "competition of the Paris cane manufacturers was unique." The horn and tortoise canes of A. Burgi were especially mentioned. I was unable to find any information with respect to Vienna or Berlin, but the court jeweler Wilm at Schinkenbruecke always used to sell gold knobs.

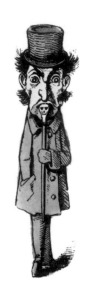

Fig. 29 Gentleman with skull cane from "Muenchner Bildrbogen" no. 18 "A gay society," circa 1850.

Doctor's canes

A golden knob decorated the cane of any successful medical doctor. During the reign of Louis XVI, doctors started carrying long canes, when going over land, as a sign of their status. In the article "The dress of the doctor over three centuries," written by Grete de Francesco and published in "Ciba Zeitschrift" in 1936, the author says: "The dress of the doctor became the fashionable dress of the bourgeois. However, several class attributes remained until the 19th century, especially the doctor's cane with the gold knob, which from region to region had its own forms and characteristics, just as much as the cane was sometimes slimmer sometimes thicker. The cane was always present, as can been seen on many contemporary prints. Even on a drawing, which shows the most famous doctor of the pre-revolution 'Tout Berlin,' the 'old Heim' working on his desk, the cane has not been missed." The old Heim, a poor mens' doctor, has a simple wooden cane, mounted with a watch. With the iron ferrule he marked those

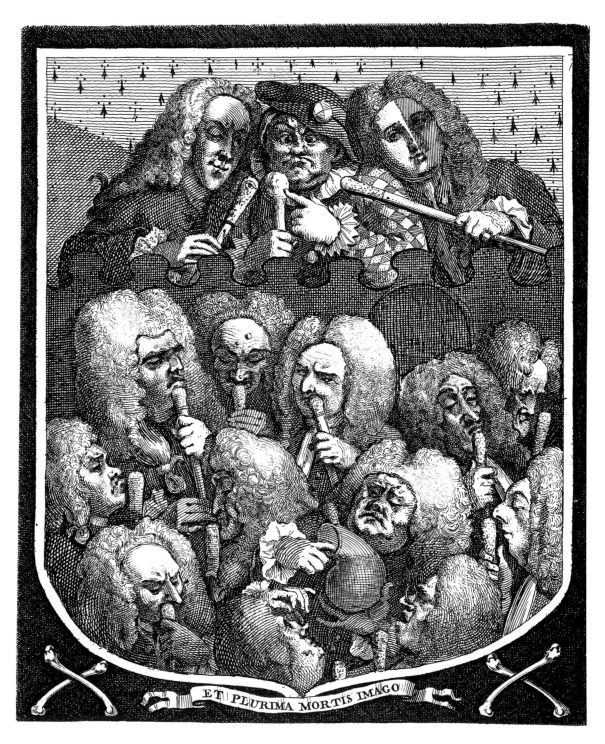

Fig. 30 The Collegium Medicum by William Hogarth,
March 1736. The text refers to "15 Quack Heads and
their 15 Cane Heads."

doors which opened only after lengthy knocking and pounding. If he went to see noble clients he would carry a spanish cane with a golden knob. He had lost at least one of these in July 1793 on his way from his apartment at the corner of Kronen and Markgrafenstrasse to Bellevue, the castle of Prince Ferdinand.

Fifteen doctors are pressing golden cane knobs against their chins and noses on the William Hogarth print "The company of Undertakers" from 1736. The knobs of doctors' canes were set with compartments for pills, or, during the late 17th and early 18th century, the pique canes contained so called "Pomander." These containers held smelling liquids such as ambra (= pomme d'ambre) and were carried on a chain. The fragrance was smelled for medical purposes, to shield against the plague. The pomander canes could be unscrewed (see illustration 326), the compartment set with a vinegar or perfume filled sponge and the vapors smelled through the little holes on the lid. Doctors also carried smelling salt to revive fainted patients.

Canes with serpents have been mentioned in the chapter about magical canes and as status canes for mayors. The cane with a serpent, however, can also be a cane representing the medical profession. These are the canes which are made either of bone or ivory with a serpent winding up or down on the cane. The comparison with the snake cane of Asklepions, the heavenly doctor of classical Greece, comes to mind, and also, that a doctor might choose the Asklpions cane as his cane. Whether the hand, holding a serpent (a rather frequent motif on canes) should also be counted as a doctor's cane was discussed by Prof. Dieter Banzhaf in two articles, but could not be decided conclusively. So far the only answer really is, that any cane worn by a medical doctor during a medical visit has to be called a doctor's cane. It is certainly easier to be specific, when talking about canes which contain medication and instruments. The encyclopedia author Krunitz writes: "canes containing surgical instruments, such as scalpel, scissors, knives, which were stored in the knob, which could be unscrewed ... the canes were usually custom-made by the same mechanic who manufactured the instruments." The most complicated cane can be seen at the "Royal College of Surgery in England" in Edinburgh, made in 1872, it is illustrated in Dike under number 23/7. Followers of the Phrenologie of Dr. F.F. Gall used a cane with an ivory knob in the form of a human head, indicating the various parts of the brain, numbered and divided into soul and spiritual areas. (see illustration 324, 325).

As a side note, I would like to mention the different handicapped canes, among which the canes with integrated hearing aide are the rarest and the most desired by collectors.

Students: "Bummlers and Ziegenhainers"

During the 18th century, the German student from Jena wore a thick cane, just like an apprentice, which he even took to lectures. The main reason lay in the vicinity or the cane producing village of Ziegenhain, which caused this fashion. Otherwise students did not wear canes yet. In a script for 1739 "Important notes from the life style at the University at Goettingen" every item which a student will need and should know is listed, including its price. The tobacco pipes, the long ones from the Netherlands, were included at 6 gr the dozen," but canes were not mentioned. The first time those can be seen in student prints is at the turn of the 19th century, very clear on the lithograph "the true student," which compares the new student to the "petit maitre" of the rococo. A young man with a beard and pipe, high boots and a knotty stick, shows off in front of a breaches and sword bearer of the past. "Caution if you get too close with your perfumed jacket. He will call you a perfume stallion, you risk getting hit with his knotted cane."

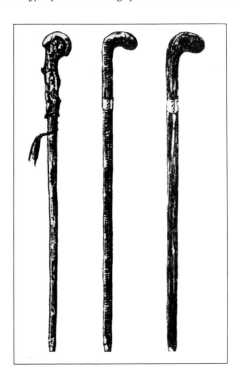

Fig. 31 Thick natural wood canes of the "Goat Herdsman Type" from the catalog of Wilhelm Schuss, 1890.

Ziegenhain, located only a few miles from Jena, was the beer town for the students. The "Ziegenhainer canes" were made there. Made from the wood of the local cherry trees, which grew around Freiburg/Unstrut, Frankenhausen and Stadtsulza, they were roasted in the oven of the brewery of Ziegenhain. They were turned until the bark fell off and the cane had the correct dark brown color. The remaining bark was removed under water. The canes were dried in the basement of the brewery. Some inhabitants of Ziegenhausen supposedly made between 500 and 600 taler per year with these canes. Later, the Ziegenhainer canes were manufactured industrially by three companies in Buergel/Thuringen.

Student canes can be easily identified, usually even dated. They were decorated with armorial crests and emblems of the fraternities, often carried the name of the owner, the donor, because, since the Biedermeier period it was custom to give presents in memory of a relationship. The "color students" had developed particular dedication gifts such as pipes, stains, silhouette portraits and canes. The most common formula was "XY s.l. LBF YZ" (= seinem lieben Leibfuchsen). Two early canes do exist. The Baggel (from Baculus) of Jeremias Gotthelf which is in the Town Museum of Zofingen, and the Ziegenhainer cane of the Frankish Fraternity, which is now owned by the Corps Franconia-Jena in Regensburg. The Gotthelf cane of the 20th and the 19th century is inscribed with symbols and names of the founding members of the Zofingia Bern. The cane of Regensburg originally belonged to the theology student Christian Dieter Schorr (his name is outstandingly decorated on it). Schorr received it from Friedrich Witter. It carries various symbols and 28 engraved names. It also has scratch marks which makes one believe that it was used in student initiations.

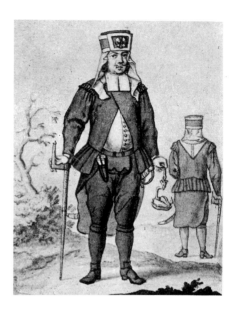

Fig. 32 The mountain costume of an Elder from the Plauenschen Grund, with red vest and gold lace on white cap and white collar. He leans against a mountain hook. From the book about costumes by Heinrich Fehlingk, 1719, at the occasion of the marriage of the Saxon Elector and the Emperor's daughter Maria Josepha.

During the middle of the nineteenth century, canes with ivory knobs became popular. The so called "bummler" with a flat knob was a fine successor of the Ziegenhainer canes. In a catalog of the company Glaser & Sohn, Dresden 1895, we can find prices: an armorial knob cane with a 20 cm ivory handle was between 40 and 45 Marks; a cane with straight handle and crest was between 30 and 35 Marks. Mounted on ebony, each of the canes cost an additional 20 Marks.

There were many different forms of walking sticks which could be identified by emblem and crest as student canes. The Baltic Corps, for example, always carried a heavy oak cane with pointed tip and crooked handle: the typical Alpine cane. Bamboo canes with silver dedications, antler handles with porcelain plates set in the rose were also used by students. A brief fashion of the 1870s brought in 50 cm long canes with an ivory disc as a knob.

Mining students from Freiburg/Sachsen are illustrated in paintings and on KPM porcelain figures wearing mountain hatchets as canes. These mountain hatchets are cane high with axe shaped handles, usually cast in brass and highly decorated. These hatchets have appeared since the 15th century and are part of the elaborate costume and rank hierarchy of mountain farming regions. Even today they are presented as honorary hatchets at special occasions. For example, the alumnus of the mining student of

Notes about mountain hatchets

the Ruhr region receive one after 50 years of work in the mining industry. These were decorated with reliefs showing their work underground, with huts, towers and mining tools.

Most of the mountain hatchets which are part of collections are from no earlier than the first decades of the twentieth century.

Hunting canes

Hunters like to wear heavy decorated weapons, and their canes also show that they are followers of Saint Hubertus. An antler's rose as a handle is the simplest form of hunting cane. The rose could be carved, as a dog's head or as game, for example. The handle made of antler could be turned into a dog whistle. The rose could be set with an armorial crest made of either silver or ivory. These works, which frequently combine hunting and riding, were usually made in Dresden, Bautzen and Gorlitz, some from Geisling and der Steige. According to the German Ivory Museum they were not made in Erbach, despite being called that in the trade. Erbach did make hunting brooches, but not cane handles.

Canes as souvenir

The souvenir is a form of social passport, a prestige object: it shows that one is well traveled. Trips to foreign countries were special, travel to exotic countries were rare. The typical regional walking cane is one of the last souvenirs which can be bought. While almost every other souvenir is marketed world wide: one has to go to Jersey to purchase a Giant Jersey Cabbage Stick, a stick made of special cabbage bearing the crest of Jersey on the handle. The same is true for a shark spine cane form the Seychelles or a Makila, the basque weapons cane, which only exists in Bayonne.

For over 100 years the classic souvenir from Ceylon and India is a walking cane with an elephant's head. It might be made of ebony and carved primitively, or a true art piece with inlaid ivory teeth. The most interesting combination which I have seen was a leather head with a soft trunk, ivory teeth, and ivory ears on a heavy dark shaft. Another typical Indian cane is the Guptis, which is a sword cane with a European blade. Usually they are made rather crudely, sometimes they are even mass produced.

The typical European souvenir canes are:

—A finely carved horse's head made of wood, "Kerkyra" carved in Greek letters. It is from Korfu, the fashionable vacation spot during the Belle Epoche, with intense social life, horse races and Wilhelm II as amateur archeologist.

—A short Scottish crook neck which ends in a stylish thistle. A modern variation has a soccer player's leg and soccer ball.

—A cane made of cork oak in the form of a closed umbrella (around 1900) from the Isle of Wight.

—Irish black thorn canes, painted black. Locals will repaint their canes every year.

—On the Greek island of Crete, shepherds' crooks are sold with stylized dolphin handles. The look is the same as it was 100 years ago.

Most of the walking canes from Africa or the South Sea were specifically made for the European tourist. Sometimes in the western style, sometimes according to tribal traditions. One can find heads with tropical helmets, or heads of natives, either naturalistic or vague. In the Republic of Ruanda and in Camerun pearl covered canes are sold (= ikoni) with round knobs and iron ferrule, which do have tribal tradition. On the African East Coast the Kamba carvers, who also carve ebony busts, create high quality canes. On the Pitcairn Islands in the Southsea, canes with stylized birds' heads are offered to tourists, and in New Zealand traces are left of the famous, highly prized Maori canes.

The contemporary Chinese canes are produced with dragons' heads motifs from the Jiangxi province or are rattan canes from Sezchuan. The canes from Shaanxi are made of wood which is polished to a glassy finish. None of these canes are spectacular and they are not always offered in the friendship stores.

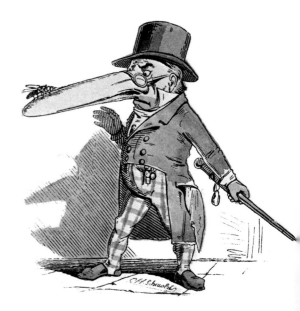

Fig. 33 Gentleman with long nose by Ch. Schmolze in "Muenchner Bilderbogen," Nr. 18, circa 1850.

Go into the forest: the cane and folk art

In the beginning there was naturally grown wood. If one needed a stick or cane, one went into the forest and searched for the right piece of wood with the perfect fork. The wood was rarely treated, the cane was not expected to last, and it was a functional piece. Some are illustrated in the catalogue of the Styrian Joanneum Museum "Wood its natural form." But pure functionalism has always been short lived with human beings: the simple stick needed to be decorated. The handle is the part most suitable for decoration. The most common motifs were human beings and animal heads. The head can be turned into a whole animal, one animal can turn into an entire scene. The form of the wood would be the inspiration for the carver. Starting at the handle, the whole cane could be covered with carving. Knots in the wood are further inspiration, and an old law of folk art says: cover empty spaces with decoration.

The comedy "Figaro in Germany" by August Wilhelm Iffland, printed in 1790, contains the character of the 58 year old Count Christoph who "goes hunting and carved canes with birds' heads."

I met a gentleman in Munich, who carves canes for pleasure and only for his own use. Mr. Sparka has told me about his work: he is the best example of a wood carver in the farmer's, shepherd's and wood worker's tradition. Besides a talent for carving, an in-depth knowledge of wood types is necessary, a sharp eye and imagination to see the future handle arise from a root. The following is Mr. Sparkas explanation:

About the Carving of Handles

"Complete" canes, shaft and handle together, are rarely found in nature, unless one cuts a tree. Such rare finds usually have a handle which is only slightly thicker than the shaft, which means it can only be carved in relief.

Wood for handles can only be found on long walks after heavy snow damage or storms or while strolling through cleared forests. After finding a suitable piece of root, one should always cut 10 cm more than necessary. Even when wood is dried and dead, when it is cut it will chip at the cut line. The best saw for a cane searcher is the double toothed one that is part of the Swiss Army Knife. Cut planes should be sealed with strong lacquer or, even better, with sticky wood amber seal, as used by gardeners. Then it should dry for a year or longer, but while exposed to the elements.

This means that the cellar is not suitable: the wood will dry to fast, which means interior cracks. In the garage there is usually not sufficient ventilation and the wood will mold.

The stored and debarked wood is covered with a clear glaze, which hinders the remaining moisture from leaving the wood too fast and increases the appearance of the wood pattern. The carving knives used should have very short blades (one to two centimeters), knives with interchangeable blades have advantages because the blades tend to break. Sandpaper is the only additional aide. Anything else would be considered sculpturing. This limits the size of my handles: it is very frustrating to work during the days before finishing the raw piece.

It is harder to find the right wood for the shaft. Fresh shafts can have light bends which can be straightened by attaching the shaft with wood screws to a straight piece of wood and letting the shaft dry for about half a year.

The most suitable woods are: white thorn and black thorn, ash, hazel and cherry, white beech, various willows, maple and chestnut, and the twigs of lime trees. If you have your own garden you may grow any wood for 5 to 10 years in a controlled manner.

Basically any wood is suitable for shafts. The best wood to start carving is from the lime tree, it is by far the softest. For a cane that is to be used it is not suitable, because the equilibrium of the cane is too low and the cane will get dents when hitting the floor. The next best wood for the beginner is ash. It can be used right away, because it does not require time to dry. The bark has to be removed at once (do not forget the glaze). Other frequently used woods are pear and cherry. Not suitable are apple and peach, since movement of the wood and inner cracks can not be avoided. Kernel cherry is so hard that the knife will frequently break, while birch and robinie will make nice handles. But, generally speaking, one does not choose the wood, but rather the form of the wood.

With respect to the creative aspect of his work, I would like to quote Mr. Sparka: "the creative work will take longer than the actual carving. Unless, of course, one is happy with copying classical motifs. These will lead to a quick success but are boring in the long run. Creating a new motif sometimes requires days or weeks with a piece of wood (glazed of course), turning it and imagining what is hidden in the piece. Possible motifs are sketched with a pen directly on the wood — often, to be removed again. As soon as the desired form is in front of the eye — which is hard for the untrained eye — the inner pictured is tested by looking at any available photographs (Mr. Sparka only carves animals). The best test is, for example, to watch a living animal in the zoo. Typical proportions and orders have to be registered. To just copy nature is not sufficient. The material and the future function of the piece (a good fit in the palm and strength) do not allow motifs such as hedgehogs and erected horses' ears. To imagine the figure in the raw wood is important for three reasons: 1. One should never change the image while carving — to change a horse into a dog will look like a bastard at the end. 2. the carving has to be done in one day — otherwise the inner image disappears and the characteristics, which one concentrates to carve, are gone. 3. Because some of the pieces do have knots, those will have to be integrated and used for eyes, mouths or ears. Eventually a harmonic figure will be created around such impurities."

Nature helps

There has always been a custom among farmers and wood workers to let sticks grow under supervision. Joseph Blau writes in "The house industry and folk art in the Bohemian Forest," Prague 1917: "A beautiful walking cane made from juniper wood needs several years of pruning and waiting. The forester chooses a promising bush, cuts the lower branches and lets it grow; the same happens the next year, the higher branches will grow stronger. The third year, the cuts are nicely made. Now the stick is cut, the bark is taken off, bent by putting it into hot water, and finished. These canes are very durable, feather weight and very pretty; but, they have to be well hidden under bushes and branches, otherwise they could be stolen by somebody else." Ritz continues by telling that during his mother's life time it was considered unethical to cut a stick that somebody else was waiting for.

In Lindewerra, a house trade of cane makers developed from 1840 onward. a vine was placed around growing wood. This "devil's vine" was so tight that it left marks on the wood. These canes were highly thought of by the students in Goettingen, who usually purchased them for the traditional Ascension Day procession. In the Swiss Emmental region the chip-carving was called "hicken," which was usually done on hazels with initials and date.

The first picture canes had religious themes. They narrated the story of the suffering of Jesus Christ or the life of the Saints. They were owned by priests, were commissioned work by an artist, and pilgrims covered their canes with the stations of their pilgrimage and with symbols of Saints. The canes were their entry pass into cloisters and hostels.

These type of canes were then also worn by farmers — which makes the dating very difficult. The figures and symbols on church benches and pulpits were models for the carvers until the 19th century.

Regional identification is very difficult. The usual attribution as "Alpine" is very often wrong, the cane might very well be from the flat lands of the Netherlands, as can be seen in the book by H. Wiegersma "Folk Art in the Netherlands." It can be said that professionally carved canes are harder to pinpoint than the primitive ones. The professional can very well produce an Alpine scene with game poacher and a milk maid despite living in the Rhine valley; the individual with leisure time he wants to use to beautify his cane is more inspired by the animals, flowers and objects of his immediate surroundings. Besides traditional carvings, the cane could be also just decorated by chip carving —a very early type of work — or by pinning. Illustration 47 shows a tattooed cane from England with fox hunting scenes. There is also a dated and attributed piece with this technique in the Bavarian National Museum: an Italian pilgrim's cane from the 17th century is entirely covered with scenes, which appear to be etched. It is definitely not folk art. There are certain similarities between these canes and the scrimshaw technique of the whalers.

Besides religious motifs (the most beautiful is a Father-thou shall be in heaven cane in a Bavarian private collection), one finds forest animals, soldier scenes, hunting scenes and mythological subjects and fairy tales which are all hard to attribute. Commemorative canes do exist; for example, the cane carved in commemoration of the Mexican-American War in 1914: it is very finely done, very naturalistic and not without humor, the American eagle has very ruffled feathers.

Common subjects are: a bearded man as the handle (the bearded man has been the sign of a humanist since the Renaissance); animal heads made of branch knots, with dramatically opened mouth; the double face, the second face can be set on the inside of the bend in the handle; the monsters, lizards and drag-

Pictorial canes

ons, which emerge from the wood; snakes, which crawl out of the cane or wind on the cane or that turn into the cane. An old reference to the possible provenance after Kruenitz: "firgural canes, which came from the Black Forest had handles carved as dogs, lions, wolves, birds, fish and other figures."

Herdsman and shepherd's canes

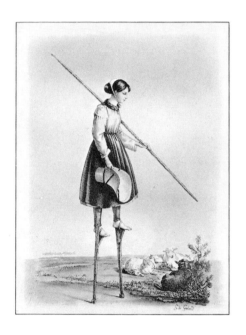

Fig. 34 Shepherd from the French Landais region on stilts and long stick. Print from 1830.

There are two terms for two related professions: the herdsman tends the cattle and pigs, the shepherd tends sheep.

If we want to have more general rules we would say: shepherds' canes are more characteristic and easier to identify than those used by herdsmen; the Scottish shepherds use neck crooks, the German shepherd uses a shovel, in Scandinavia and Switzerland a ring cane is used, iron rings are attached to a stick; Greek canes are easily identified.

Besides the working cane, shepherds often wore a highly decorated cane as part of their costume — a holy day cane. Hungarian herdsmen and shepherds are good examples to study, their canes also characterize their specialization, are well documented and researched, and are found in museum collections.

The following cane types are known: straight staffs without handles with decorative and figural tin or bone inlay for all herdsmen, but especially the ones tending horses; knot sticks for cattle decorated with chip carving, the chips colored with pigment or wax; hatchet sticks for the pig herdsmen (the metal part, sometimes decorated, is the handle); and heavily decorated shepherd's staffs with crook handle. The ram's head is on almost every single one. One can almost identify carving and artist schools, the good pieces were used as models for other generations.

The canes of prisoners and soldiers

Illustration 231 shows a cane decorated with straw. The technique of straw marquetry, a fine and unusual type of inlay, was developed and exclusively produced by French prisoners in England during the Napoleonic Wars (1793-1815). There were 6000 prisoners in the Norman Cross Camp, Huntingdonshire, held for many years. Similar to shepherds, whalers and seamen, some sort of trade was necessary. Under the guidance of professionals (Napoleon's army had been recruited from all levels of the working population), famous ships made of bone, bone chests and boxes, bangles and cane handles were made, which can easily be confused with the works of seamen.

Chest, tea caddies, fans and canes were inlaid with straw. The technique is as follows: flawless straws were cut into 8 inch long pieces and cut in half length-wise, quarters, eighths and sixteenths. The small straw pieces were then colored. The original claim that the colors were achieved with teas is wrong; first of all the range of the colors is much too wide and, second, tea was not available to prisoners of war. The marquetry maker arranged the straws by color, painted a sketch on thin paper, glued the straw pieces, which were cut to size, on the paper. Glue was made by boiling bones. The chest, or for our example the cane, was covered with heavier brown paper, which was covered with glue and the straw paper was then attached. When holding the cane in hand one would not believe the simplicity of the technique and one has to admire the delicate finger work.

Prisoners of war also made carved canes, which are harder to identify, unless dated or inscribed, which was quite common. The thoughts about life in freedom are reflected, and many of these canes have erotic themes.

Canes decorated with the German eagle or a swastika were never made by prisoners. This would not have been tolerated by the guards. These either simple or more elaborate canes, inscribed "Leningrad" or "Wolchow" are the canes actually used in mud covered trenches. Canes decorated with snakes might have been worn by the First Aid and Medical personnel, which had to move around a lot in muddy territory. The swastika has been removed on many of these canes after the end of the war.

Carpenter Canes and other guild customs

Once in a while carpenters from Hamburg can be seen wearing their large black hats, the wide corduroy pants and the heavy, turned walking sticks called "Stenz." Until three years ago Master Egle has hand-made these carpenter canes, sketched on a piece of ash and carving the turns with a rasp. The cane was closely tied to the customs of the carpenters. When a wandering carpenter entered a hostel, he had to button the cane underneath his jacket in such a way that only a short piece would stick out. When settling in the hostel the cane and tool had to be placed under the table and covered with a large, red handkerchief. Because the cane was considered a dangerous weapon, it had to, when entering a village, be carried horizontally, covered by the other tool, which was carried on the back. Several conflicts were reported in Berlin in the middle of the 19th century because pedestrians were bothered by the cane. Because the guild wanted to continue the cane tradition, carpenters were no longer allowed to use the sidewalk.

By tradition, any unmarried craftsman had to wander and could not settle, and so the hand cane was important. The turners usually had very elaborate ones, the masons carried canes similar to the carpenters, and the cabinet makers used a cane which also served as a measure. The stone masons had a bamboo cane with a silver knob, which they carried in both hands, diagonally across the breast, left hand above the right hand, when entering another stone masons atelier, according to Carl Heimsch in 1872.

These wandering canes later became the fraternity and guild canes, a relic of which is still carried in Corpus Christi day precession and can be found in some churches. The book "Stanglsitzerheilige und Grosse Kerzen" by the Finkenstaedts (1968) lists over 2000 examples in Upper Bavaria, Schaben, Lower Bavaria and Upper Pfalz, including guild staffs of all trades, including ship makers and operators.

In France, the "compagnons" canes carried by the member of "compagnonnages," which include many different guilds organized by trade and region. The ferrules are characteristically either short for the road or long for ceremonial occasions. In addition, the canes were decorated with ribbons. The colors correspond with the colors of the guild, worn by the apprentices that left a place to start their journey and who were accompanied by their fellow workers out of town. The cane knob has a medallion carrying the name of the owner, the date when entering the guild and the emblems of the guild, which usually included the typical tools of the trade. The canes could be short or long. Some appear harmless, others had iron, copper or brass decorations and looked like weapons.

The cane shafts usually made of whale bones and the handles of whale teeth. They tell the tale of patient and simple minds. They are a testament to the poetry and the sometimes unbelievable artistry of these seamen. That some of those pieces of art were made with simple knives, improvised files and chisels, which were nothing but nails, explains Herman Melville's lines in "Moby Dick." "Whoever is damned to life far from the Christian world will inevitably sink back into the style that he was saved from by the Lord: he will turn again into a savage. A true whaler is a savage like an Iroquois. I am also one. The only King I accept is the one of cannibalism, and this only as long as it pleases me. One of the most characteristic trade marks of these savages is their patience which is developed with small crafts. An old battle club, an old spear tip from Hawaii are true triumphs of human patience, comparable to a Latin dictionary. Over the course of many years a piece of shell, or a piece of whale tooth is used to carve an intricate interwoven pattern into the weapon. As patient as his Hawaiian brother is the white savage, the seaman. With the same patience he guides his knife, his one and only, or his shark tooth. The pieces he makes are densely covered with patterns, barbaric, thoughtful and touching, comparable to the wood cuts of Albrecht Duerer, the wild German."

The jaw bone of the grey whale were to most treasured ones. Besides "Moby Dick" the tools of the seamen were also described in the log book of the "Grace," which was kept in 1912 and 1913 and which describes small work benches which were used for manufacturing canes on still days. This explains the turned columns on the canes seen in illustration 78. The same log book talks about how men used the polished spines of sharks on iron rods for walking canes. In "The cruise of the Cachalot," Frank T. Bullen writes in 1899 that a good carver and scrimshaw maker could produce about one dozen canes on one trip. Scrimshaw is the term used in New England for any work by a whaler made from fish bone, whale bone and the teeth of whales and/or walrus. The material had to be used shortly after the catch, otherwise it became too dry.

The primitive decorative carvings which were done on whales teeth are now typically referred to as scrimshaw. After the etching, the lines are stained with ink or soot. Illustration 70 shows a handle with a whaling scene. This cane and some others are from the Calhoun collection of "Yankee Whaler's Scrimshaw." Origi-

The canes of seamen and whalers

nally part of the Butt & Smith Whale Craft Collection, they are mostly from the middle and the second half of the 19th century. Especially with respect to teeth, the provenance is very important, because there are many forgeries. On the other hand, the whaling fleet of the United States had about 700 ships in 1850.

Sperm whale teeth and walrus teeth with ivory handles were carved as decorative knots (reminiscent of a turkish turban), as column capitals, as hands, ladies legs, dice, buttons, whales and birds. The bone shafts were carved in fish skin patterns, with tile patterns, spirals or striations, and were inlaid with ebony, tortoise, horn or fish bone. Different patinas ranging from warm brown and honey yellow to patterned white offer an aesthetic appearance, underscored by their romantic provenance.

The amazing world of system canes

Ever since man used a cane, inventors and fuss pots have given canes additional functions. They either added a feature to the cane or they hid something in the shaft or handle. If one believes the Greek mythology, Prometheus was the first system cane maker. "He lit his torch on the fiery wagon of the sun, broke off a piece of coal and pushed it into the cavity of the stem of a giant funnel, blew out his torch and disappeared. This is the way mankind received fire." (Servius about Virgil's Ecloga). The next use of a system cane can not be proven either, one has to just believe it: the first silk worm cocoons were smuggled by pilgrims from China to Byzanz in the cavities of canes.

Craftsmen made complicated canes over centuries for noble gentlemen, which are described in inventories and museum collections. The palace museum of Greenwich describes a cane owned by Henry VIII which contained a set of tools in its handle: pliers, a tape measure, a knife, a file and a gold set stone. In addition, it held a perfume flask, a sundial and a compass.

Multi-purpose canes continued to be made when cane production was industrialized during the second half of the 19th century. Illustrations 260-264 show a cane from an English collection: It is probably the most complex system cane ever made, a unique piece, custom-made for a crazy client.

What are system canes?

A cane with a double function is still offered today: the umbrella cane. There are two basic models. One has an umbrella attached to the handle, and when using the umbrella the shaft is unscrewed and folded and carried in the coat pocket. The other one has an umbrella with the handle inside the shaft of the cane, which is taken out and used, while the cane does not use its function. Many different models were popular, but the umbrella cane had its real breakthrough after Samuel Fox in 1852 replaced the crude fish bone umbrella rods with thin metal ones. The silk cover also had to be as thin as possible. The Hugendubel company in Stuttgart claimed in the 1920s to be "the inventor of umbrella canes." In 1929 97 companies producing umbrella canes were registered in the German Reich. An umbrella cane is a good example for the two most important characteristics of a system cane: it wants to hide something, or it want to combine several things or functions. At a time when everybody was carrying a cane it could

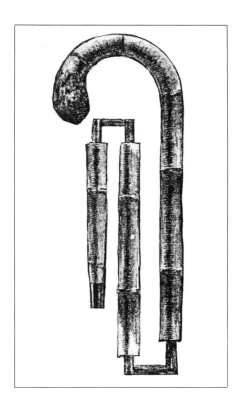

Fig. 35 Folding cane for traveling. Folding canes are still made today. From "Pearson's Magazine," July 1897.

be used to carry something useful or useless along. It seems to be a remote cousin of the briefcase, which later pushed the cane aside. The piano tuner carried his hammer, the smoker his cigarette, the lady her toiletry, the horse trader his shoulder gauge, the gentleman a gold pen or change and the photographer carried his tripod in the cane.

With respect to the terminology of these multi-purpose canes: the most correct is the term system cane, which corresponds to the French canne a systeme. The more romantic terms, such as a cane with an inner life or a cane with soul, are similar to the Italian baston con anima. In English speaking countries the hidden aspect is stressed, by referring to it as a secret cane or to the surprise effect when calling it a gadget cane.

Over 1500 patents have been issued for these cane, and many more have been built and invented, without being patented. In the book "Les Cannes a Systeme" by Catherine Dike one can find an almost complete catalogue of system canes. More than 1600 canes have been identified and photographed, the register contains 500 terms for objects, from Acethylen lamp to zither, which are built into canes or used as canes. I would like to focus on a few special areas of system canes, which will also be illustrated, to give a clear picture to the reader. I will bring some additions to the work of Catherine Dike for the collector.

Different types of system canes

The wide range of system canes can be brought into some order — in basic categories and not just groups of canes. The first category encompasses professional canes which have a real purpose. The tuning fork helps the musician to tune his instrument. Wine salesmen had canes (German patent 1887; French patent 1903) which could suck liquids from a glass into the cane. It seems like the glass had been drunk, while indeed the wine was stored in the cane to be released outside before visiting the next client. Never patented, this useful cane was well described in the diary of the Munich Brewer Gabriel Sedlmayr, which he kept during an England trip in 1833. Sedlmayr was anxious to learn the secrets of English brewing and tried to get samples of the fermenting product, to test and measure back in his hotel. However, it turned out to be impossible to fill the liquids in little bottles without detection. "In order to avoid that, we had little canes made, which were lacquered metal with a valve at the bottom, allowing the cane to be filled when submerged in beer, but when lifted the valve would close, holding the liquid in the cane, which allows us to steal safely." It worked well, only one brewery noticed the act "Fatal discovery of unfair means."

The fabric merchants, shoe makers and the coffin makers carried their measures in their canes, the surveyor carried a tripod, and the cheese maker a little screw driver, to name but a few.

The second category is composed of the so called practical canes, which are aides for hikers and hunters or help with other outdoor occupations. The umbrella canes are part of this category, the cane containing a pipe and tobacco in the shaft (sold by Dunhill at present), the cane with a candle and flash light to read house numbers in the dark; various seat canes, the cane with dog whistle and game call; the tourist cane with a cap in the handle, a shaving kit and a tooth brush; canes with fishing rods and butterfly net, canes with binoculars or a secret camera, with dice or musical instruments. Some of those "practical" canes are also part of the next category, these are canes containing gadgets or other unusual surprises. Automatons, figural handles which turn and blink the eyes, move their tongue (see later discussion), water spouting canes, usually as silver Chinese, with a movable ponytail as a handle. Canes with hidden erotic scenes. Looking glasses, where one sees an image when looking though a small hole. The most sophisticated one of these contained a show of up to 30 slide, patented in France under "canne merveilleuse." It contained slides of either landscapes or erotic scenes. I would also like to include cigarette and cigar holders in this category, smoking from a quail's head or a clown's head attracts a lot of attention.

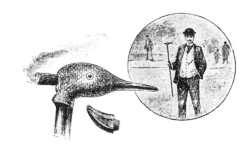

Fig. 36 Cane with cigarette holder in the form of a partridge head. From "Pearson's Magazine," July 1897.

Curiosities and oddities

In the fourth category are canes with integrated instruments to measure distance (pedometers) or time (watches) or to do other examinations (microscopes, lupe), unless these were already in one of the previous categories.

One has to understand that even at the end of the nineteenth century, during the high period for system canes, these were neither common nor widely used canes. They were always prestige objects (both in their capacities as curiosities and when they were used as professional canes), as one can see from contemporary magazines. The article in "Peason's Magazine" from July 1897 is called "Walking Stick Wonderland" and reflects the amazement about these canes as does the cane exhibition in Paris 1980 *Le monde inconnu des cannes*. The exhibition raised a world wide nostalgia and amazement about the past while the article showed, through many illustrations, which types of canes did exist: the cane as cigar holder, as telescope, as parcel carrier, as horse measure, for the doctor fitted with medicine bottles, scissors, scalpel, and injection needles; for a geologist with compartments for stone samples and a hammer; the folding cane for traveling, the writing tools, the drinking beaker; with comb and brush; with knife, fork and cork screw; as pistol, as folding table, with cigarette case; as color and brush container; as match boxes; as candle stick holder and as life savers. The latter cane contains a strong balloon, which can be pulled from the cane, inflated and attached to the cane. It was meant as a life saver from drowning. It is similar to the florists cane, patented in Germany in 1877, which contains a compass, a gardener knife, thermometer, hour glass and a flute, to call for help after falling into a canyon. System canes are full of oddities.

There are still system cane inventors among us. Over the last few years three different canes received patents for the removal of dog stool, sealing them in a container for temporary storage.

Notes to the cane collector: system canes rarely are attractive on the outside, they are either functional or intentionally simple in appearance. Straight canes with multiple inner lives do not want to attract attention. This explains why many of them were not kept after the owner passed away, they were either removed or banished to the attic. There they were found by children, their secrets were detected and their content was dispersed, broken or lost. Therefore complete system canes are rare, the rarer the richer the insides. This is reflected at auctions and through auction results.

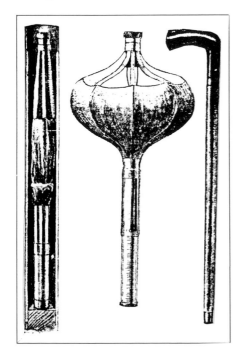

Fig. 37 An inflatable life saver. From "Peason's Magazine," July 1897.

In his encyclopedia about the "walking stick," Johann Georg Kunitz uses three pages to explain the pace maker: "which is a cane used for walking that has a machine attached which counts the steps." A flexible ferrule transmitted every pushing of the cane to a counting machine.

The first pedometers were made around 1730. The pedometers described by Max von Boehn in the Mathematischen Salon in Dresden, the oldest of which was the "Lehmann Reinharz" signed and dating from 1740, do not exist anymore; they were destroyed during the Second World War.

Sun dials were early time keepers, such as the valuable model in the possession of Count Albrecht of Bavaria (Illustration 297). A Verge Watch is set in the cane of Maximilian III of Bavaria (Illustration 295, 296). During the 17th and 18th century, pocket watches were built into the handles of canes, a luxury reserved for very wealthy people.

The most suitable watch movement was the Verge escapement since it was wound and set from the front. But higher grade movements, such as the cylinder and lever escapements were never made for canes. Special winding mechanisms were patented: 1. winding by turning the upper part of the watch (Swiss patent 1888). 2. The watch is wound with a crown hidden on the side of the cane (Swiss patent 1899). In all the watches with normal movement and winding mechanisms adjusted to the cane, the watch is the knob, the dial faces upwards and is open faced or covered by a lid.

The only watch movement exclusively made for a cane is the Holuska watch (Viennese patent 1885). The rectangular movement is hidden in the shaft, has a thick balance wheel, cylinder escapement which is wound by the handle. The dial is small and visible on the handle or shaft (illustration 298, 299, 300, 301). Some canes have handles with openings, where pocket watches can be carried.

Pace counters and watch canes

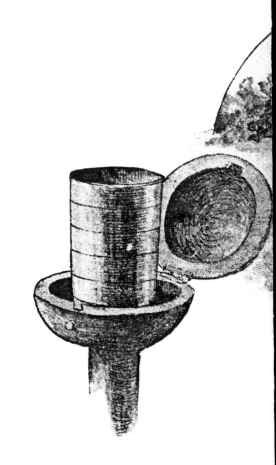

Fig. 38 When the walking stick handle contains a drinking beaker, one can drink on every spring. From "Peason's Magazine," July 1897.

Cheers with the cane

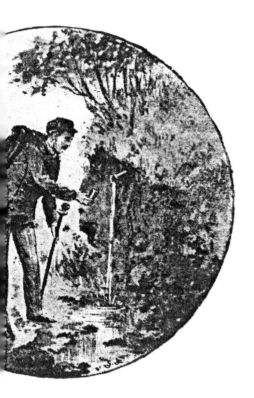

At the occasion of the wedding of Lady Di and Prince Charles, among the many souvenir items offered one could also find a drinking cane with long silver handle which contained a bottle and glass and had a medallion portrait of the couple for decoration. In the year before, the whiskey manufacturer Haig offered a drinking cane containing its noble brand Dimple: the edition size of 2978 pieces was sold out immediately.

The first drinking cane had been patented for Mr. Martin and was shown at the Industrial Fair in London 1851. Because at the time trains did not have restaurant wagons, the cane was made for the rail road traveler to quench their thirst. However, another group of users made this system cane a success. The most famous was the dwarf alcoholic painter Toulouse Lautrec, who always carried a drinking cane, resulting in the cane being called the "Toulouse Lautrec." The master's cane, which could hold half a liter of "green fee" (= absinth), his favorite drink, is exhibited in the Musee Toulouse Lautrec in Albi.

Between 1870 and 1914 a large number of these canes with bottles and glasses were made: most of them in a very crude way, with copper colored, short aluminum threads and out of metal which was painted to imitate wood. The models made of expensive woods, with cut glass and silver handles, used by gentlemen to lean against while flirting with the ballet girls and drinking a glass of cognac, were rare.

The second revival of drinking canes came during the 1920s, when these canes were made in Europe for America during the Prohibition period, when the drinking of alcohol was prohibited. In 1929, the "register for umbrella and cane makers" lists 12 companies specializing in drinking canes. The Viennese journalist Keno Knoeble recently acquired a large group of drinking canes from the inventory of the Austrian Cane Manufacturer Lischka, which had been made for the American market, but after the end of the prohibition in 1933 were not shipped. In the magazine "Collector's Journal" April 1979, he lists the different types: with one glass container and one drinking glass; with two or three glass containers for different kinds of schnapps; with one glass container and glasses for two; some also contain flashlights; very rare are additional whistles, to warn fellow drinkers in the speakeasies of approaching policemen.

Automatons are the type of cane which fascinate me most. For example, the ivory cockatoos (illustration 149) who at the push of a button opens his beak, croaks and ruffles his head feathers. He was sold by Briggs, as were the duck (illustration 203) and the Long Peak (illustration 143). Upon inquiry at Swaine Adeney Brigg and Sons, Mister R.E.J. Adeney informed me that he still remembers the automated ducks, donkeys, cats, various dogs and birds. He knows that the handles were made until the First World War exclusively for Briggs by a company in Austria; however, he did not remember the name. When Briggs turned to the company after the end of the war, the owner had died and the company had been dissolved. Since then, these canes, for which Briggs had the exclusive rights in England and from where they sold them all over the world, have not been made anymore.

These novelty canes were very expensive, costing between 30 and 40 pounds, which was a lot of money at the time. What could have motivated a gentleman to purchase a donkey which could raise its ears and open its mouth, or a monkey that could roll its eyes and stick out its tongue? For children these canes are sheer pleasure, but who would buy such an expensive item to please his children or grandchildren? Another explanation, of course, is to catch a lady's attention and start flirting. But to stick out the tongue is not the proper approach for that either. I think that the automaton canes, similar to today's pens with integrated digital watches, were purchased to please the child in every man.

German patent Nr. 23871 dates from March 8, 1883 and protects a "Cane handle with movable parts" by Ernst Bolle in Berlin. It has a skull whose "eyes, tongue and jaw" are automated by push button. The illustrated mechanism is very complicated. This skull is probably the most common automaton cane. It might have been used by wealthy medical students for numerous pranks. Wooden automaton canes, as for example the cat in illustration 169, are well carved and are similar to Viennese bronzes.

Cockatoos who ruffle their feathers

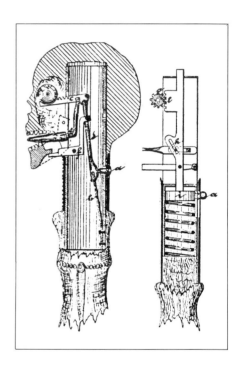

Fig. 39 Construction drawing of the patent by Ernst Bolle, 1883, as described in the text. A strong spring moves eyes, tongue and jaw via a rachet bar.

Emanuel Winternitz writes in his book "The most beautiful musical instruments of the West" "... musical instruments made in the form of walking sticks were very popular in Germany from the last decades of the 18th century to the Beidermeier. During this sentimental period the instruments which allowed the stroll-

From flute to violin: Instrument canes

ing musician to react to experiences in nature or the nightly whispering of trees or the song of the nightingale instantaneously and to express his feelings in music." This helps understand the third rhyme of the poem "The little ship" by Ludweig Uhland, from 1810. The text of the whole poem is:

Ein Schifflein ziehet leise
Den Strom hin seine Gleise
Es schweigen, die drin wandern,
Denn keiner kennt den andern.

Was zieht hier aus dem Felle
Der braune Waidgeselle?
Ein Horn, das sanft erschallet;
Das Ufer wiederhallet.

Von seinem Wanderstabe
Schraubt jener Stift und Habe
und mischt mit Flötentönen
Sich in des Hornes Dröhnen.

The wanderer described in the poem has a flute cane. Flute canes were not invented in the Biedermeier. As described by Hermann Moeck in his study about "instrument canes," the inventory of Henry VIII lists a German flute in a walking stick. And Christoh Weigel writes in 1698 in "Abbildung der Geimein-Nuetzlichen Hauptstande" about "particular walking sticks which can also be used as flutes." The musical instrument maker George Brown in Dublin ran the following advertisement on January 16, 1747 in the "Dublin Courant": "excellent German flute canes for the convenience of the gentleman who wants to relax in nature." The most famous instrument cane maker, who, in addition to flutes, clarinets and bassoons, set binoculars and smoking pipes in canes, was Ulrich Amann in Switzerland. He lived from 1766 until 1842.

Another kind of musical cane is the trumpet cane. Its handle and shaft are removed and replaced with a mouth piece and funnel. The horn cane in the "Musee du Conservatoire National de Musique" in Paris (the handle holds the mouth and resonance piece, the curved cane has double the length of the stick), and the four sided zither cane in Prague.

A cane with an integrated German flute became fashionable around 1800 and was called Czakan. The Czakan, well described in Hermann Moecks article "Czakane, Englishe und Wiener Flageolette," comes from Hungary and Slovakia and was very popular in Vienna as an amateur instrument. The cane has a crooked handle, and has its origin in the Czakany, which is an axe form weapon worn as a walking stick, which later was worn by the pig herdsmen in the Bakony forest. The long Czakan-flute cane is the forerunner of the shorter German flute, which originally was called a flute cane, which can lead to confusion, because it was also, besides the guitar, the instrument for the ramblers movement.

The harmonica cane in illustration 278 has the axe form in common with the Czakan but as a musical cane they are not related. A novelty instrument is the "Tourist Polyphon," which is a walking stick with a nickel metal handle, with ten rectangular openings. A harmonica could slide into the handle. It was by far the cheapest instrument cane. In 1901 a dozen could be bought for 20 marks or 25 franks.

The violin cane had been invented by the imperial Russian, Bavarian born court musician Johann Wilde. It has its origin in the Pochette, the narrow dance master's violin. In the "Musical News and Notes about the Year 1779," Wilde is mentioned, "I would like to mention only the most elegant pieces of his curious inventions, which he conceived and made himself. 1. a walking stick of average diameter, about 1 1/2 Zoll at the top, and which hides a violin with four strings, which has a strong tone just as any other fiddle, especially if, while playing the instrument, one leans it against another larger instrument. The plain ferrule is made of a brass ring, which can be opened to remove the bow from the shaft. A ring at the handle holds a key, similar to a watch key, which can be used to turn the four metal keys, which substitute for the peg of the violin ..." The tau-form handle is the chin piece, the bridge is lifted into place. Violin canes were made up to the first half of the nineteenth century.

In 1880, when one of the original instruments by Wilde was found, the Lutz company of Vienna copied it and offered a few for sale in 1882.

The patent 78068 for the "invention" of a "string instrument made into a walking cane" by Alexander Opikthin in St. Petersburg from 1894 is actually a replica of the old violin cane.

Fig. 40 The different ways to hold fencing canes: low, high and bent down. From Jacob Happels "Geraethfechten," 1877.

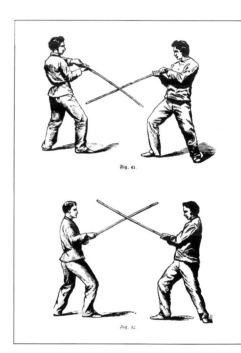

The cane as weapon

"There is no harder, meaner weapon, than a good stick in the hands of a man, who knows how to make use of it. If armed with such a weapon, a man can defend himself without fear against several attackers, whether they are carrying swords, knives or other hand arms, he can also defend himself successfully against a dangerous animal which wants to attack him." These are the introductory words by Dr. Fernand Lagrange in the book "L'Art de la Boxe francaise et de la Canne" by J. Charlemonte.

And indeed, a strong and flexible cane is an excellent weapon. If one is trained in stick fighting and self defense, one realizes that most of the weapon canes are useless inventions by the manufacturers or maliciously aggressive assault weapons because weapon canes are always concealed weapons. In order to be used as defensive weapons, the cane has to be prepared for use: the sword has to be pulled from the shaft. The "Lifesaver" with its integrated cane has to be unlocked, pulled, and one does not use the whole length of the outer cane, but gives up the range of the cane. The flails and whips have to be pulled first from the shaft, and the user of the lead weighted wires has to be properly trained. The only advantage which the sword cane has over a normal walking stick as a defensive weapon is in the tip and the deterring effect of iron. The disadvantages: one has to first pull the sword, which is harder the longer the blade, and one can not make strong blows. But the joy of invention and construction has led to many different canes with hidden weapons for hitting, pushing and shooting which, however, are prohibited from purchase, sale, or ownership. The illustrated canes in this book are exclusively in English, Swiss and French collections.

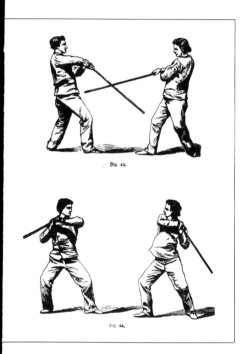

Fig 43.

Fig. 44.

The forbidden objects of the German weapons law

The Weapons Law of September 19, 1972 lists the following forbidden items: "1. Shooting instruments which are made to simulate another object of daily use" (and the other relevant chapter), "5. Cut and Thrust weapons which are made to simulate another object of daily use," and because "7. Steel rods, cudgel and brass knuckles" are also forbidden, any kind of weapons canes is illegal in Germany.

The police can "secure the object," "confiscate it," the purchaser, seller and owner can be punished with "prison to a maximum of 3 years or a monetary fine." Exemptions can be given by the Federal police.

Dukes, always concerned about their lives, were the first ones to order canes which contained swords and daggers. This had during a time when everybody was armed. With a certain surprise effect, the presumed unarmed Duke could suddenly pull a sword against his attackers. The pilgrims of the Middle Ages were in a different situation. They were not allowed to carry weapons, but were always exposed to robberies on unsafe roads. While the pilgrims' weapon cane is only known from illustrations and we can only assume from their form that they contained swords and daggers, several collections contained royal canes and references in books. The Wallace collection includes a combination sword and pistol cane. It was made in the middle of the 16th century in an atelier in Augsburg. Other known makers were the blade smith Juan Matinez, Thomas de Aiala and Francisco Ruiz in Toledo and Heinrich Col and Peter Munsten in Solingen, who used the "Passauer Wolf" as a hallmark, which originally was used by the Passau ateliers. A gun maker from Dresden has made a long dagger cane for Elector August of Saxon with an etched blade. Arch Duke Ferdinand of Tyrol had a cane with a double weapon, a Spanish dagger which contained a knife in the knob. It was part of his estate in 1596.

During the 17th century, low class people and people with bad intentions carried daggers hidden in canes, otherwise daggers were carried openly as part of the outfit. There were special daggers for promenading and walking, they were short with short handles, which were worn at peaceful occasions. Men had to carry weapons even if they were ineffective. During that period (1661), France had imposed a law against "epees en baton." The true sword canes became popular during the last third of the 18th century, when the sword as part of a man's outfit disappeared. These early sword canes, usually with ivory knobs on malacca shafts, are very rare. During the 19th century, sword canes became more and more popular and covered many pages in cane makers' catalogues. A "yellow Japanese pepper cane with an ivory hook, nickeled wired knot, Toledo Sword and feather, and a nickeled ferrule" was offered or a simple cane with an anonymous blade.

The first people to wear these sword canes were members of the military or marines. The blued steel blades with etchings, made in Solingen, were very popular. Most were made by the Runkel Company, which controlled to market world-wide. Other popular blades were made in Toledo, which always are marked in a

Sword canes:
weapon for dukes and pilgrims

Fig. 41 The air gun with all its attachment, as described on page 67, in the catalogue by W.J. George in Dover, 1899. A similar, but older model is shown in illustration 311.

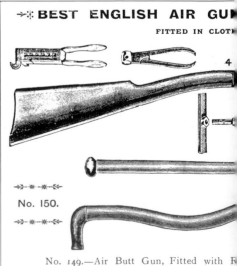

➤ BEST ENGLISH AIR GUN

FITTED IN CLOTH

No. 150.

No. 149.—Air Butt Gun, Fitted with R Times with One Charging of Air, complete w Rod, etc., £5 : 17 : 6.

No. 150.—Ditto, Air Cane, £4 : 7 : 6.

No. 151.—Ditto, but Fitted only with Ri

particular way: the Toledo name is framed by a floral design. The French blade makers were working in St. Etienne; in England in was the Wilkinson Company in London. Wilkinsons celebrated Sword Sticks were offered with a gold band and a gold knob in a light, straight antler handle. According to Pearson's magazine (1897), the English did not like swords canes very much. In France, Germany and the United States, however, they were very popular. Around the turn of the twentieth century, 19 swords cane manufacturers were working in Germany.

The swords are either double bladed with a slim edge or four six or eight sided with pointed tips. Sword canes are not often found with hollow handles and pierced decorations, some times with single bladed swords. A number of swords have protective hand pieces which are spring released. The spring is released with a push button, which holds the handle and shaft of most sword canes together. Some do have different mechanics. Catherine Dike shows, including the fire arms, a total of 385 illustrations in her book.

Swords canes are often made of bamboo, since it is hollow by nature, the most beautiful ones are made of malacca cane. Frequently, metal canes are painted or printed to simulate wood. Usually the simple cane will have a nice blade, rather than the cane with the decorated handle. The weapon should be inconspicuous. This is the reason for many of the remounts: good blades are expected to be in beautiful canes.

Daggers are either shortened swords which have been trimmed to short weapons (which can be seen on the disrupted etchings or the cut), or be made as short pieces. Daggers have to advantage of being pulled to faster. Even more effective are knives which jump out of the handle once a small cap is opened or flick knives which flicks out of the handle or shaft at the push of a button. They can be either daggers, or four sided knives.

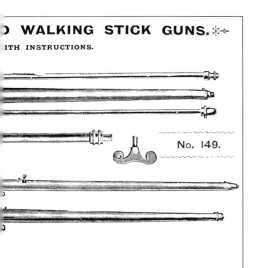

WALKING STICK GUNS. ✳←

ITH INSTRUCTIONS.

No. 149.

hot Barrels, Strong Pump, etc., will Fire Twelve
Cutter, Bullet Mould, and Shot Measure, Ram

t Barrel, £3 : 5 : 0.

A small, innocent looking cane with a Swiss/French patent and the female name "La redoubtable" (= The terrible one), or "La diabolique (= the satanic one), or "La terrible" (= the awful one) was meant as a defensive weapon. By pulling, two rows of razor blades or iron thorns cover the shaft. Instructions: "Imagine an aggressor, who wants to take your cane to deprive you of your defense. By grabbing your cane he actually activates the mechanism of the blade and will cut his hand or hands." An iron bar which is set all over with thorns is part of a Swiss collection. It can be pulled from the shaft. However, this object is just as dangerous for the owner to use than it is for the attacker. As is the lady's cane with the simple elegant metal knob, which releases six sharp blades at the push of a button and turns into a "morning star." The lady's canes with spray containers releasing sulfuric acid were also considered weapons canes. There were very un-lady like ways to harm rivals and men, which was very popular about 100 years ago. The container for the acid had to be made of glass or rubber, the tube was made of lead, since sulfuric acid will destroy almost all organic fabrics and most metals. Most of these canes were actually made for perfume or water and were used as gadget canes, and not as weapon canes. A "flagellant cane" is a cane which has wires and lead balls inside. The French patent from 1885 is more curious than effective. As discussed earlier, it is very time consuming to get the cane ready for use. Also the cudgels and club canes with lead filled handles, bronze balls or attached iron balls are useful weapons, but because of their weight and imbalance they are rather uncomfortable as walking sticks.

Funny and clever weapons

The gun cane, which John Day had patented in 1823 under number 4861, made gun history because the patent description showed the use of copper percussion caps. The weapon had a simple but reliable percussion lock, against which hammers struck from underneath. This gun was made until 1860. Its predecessors were the stone lock pistols made by Price in London, which could also be found in combination with a sword, similar to the combination weapons by William van der Kleft, who had his stone key pistol with binocular combination patented in 1814 under the patent number 3837. The weapons are signed Kleft Inventor.

Cane that can shoot

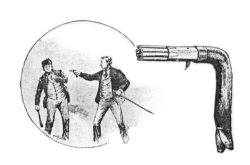

Fig. 42 The cane handle hold a multi-barrel, usually seven, pistol. This pepperbox is fired by percussion ignition. From "Pearson's Magazine," July 1897.

The earliest shooting canes were the ducal sword canes with wheel key pistols under the handle, the barrel of which was set along the blade. They are rarer than the normal wheel key weapons and are always well executed. Simpler canes were made around the middle of the 18th century; as was customary, they have stone locks. They were replaced by the percussion locks, which usually have hammers set into the handle. Only very few actually look like walking sticks, the weapon's character was obvious. With such an illegal gun cane, Louis d'Aliboud attacked the umbrella bearing Louis Philippe. He shot at the royal coach on June 25, 1836 but only hit the window frame.

In 1859 Eliphalet Remington started the serial production of a cane shotgun which had been patented by F.J. Thomas (New York) in 1859 under number 19328. It was also a percussion gun, but with a modern ignition, which made the weapon look like a walking stick. The shaft is covered with gutta-percha, a leather-like product of tree sap from the Sunfa islands. The canes had straight, slightly curved handles with eagles' claws on ball knobs. In the late 1860s, a small dog's head appeared as a handle. It took over 20 years before a breech loader gun set in a cane was made, which became the most popular American model. Cane weapons were freely developed in the United States, because contrary to Europe, poaching does not exist in the U.S. and these weapons were never outlawed. They were meant as a "protection against dogs and vagrancy."

From 1850 until 1900 hundreds of different gun cane patents were filed and in the following thirty years another 50. German gun canes did not bear the maker's name. They were considered poacher's weapons and were custom-made by the gun makers.

An unusual weapon is the cheroot gun (= the cigar gun), which has a small brass cannon as the handle. It was fired as a front loader with powder and ball and lit with the fire of a burning cigar, a deceptive weapon of the gamblers on the Mississippi river boats. One could also just fire salutes by deleting the lead.

Walking sticks with integrated revolvers with up to 40 shots were made, as well as air guns, which appear like walking canes. However, these air guns were large and heavy walking sticks, which were hard to use. After putting them under pressure with an air pump, they could fire up to 20 shots.

The art of stick fencing was taught in France during the last century. The Brevet de Cannes, color full and hand colored diplomas were given after a fencing match and were signed by witnesses. They usually show fencing scenes with neutral spectators, witnesses and watchers, mainly in military uniform. There were many fencing colleges and teachers, the rules were a combination of sword, fencing, and cane specific techniques, such as circling. In the "rose couverte," the cane was circled over the head at great speed, protecting the head like a helmet. Figures 40, 44 are the only entries to the subject in a German book "The fencing instrument" by Jacob Happel, published in 1877 in Antwerp. A good cane fencer could land between 170 and 180 blows per minute, speed and elegance were the characteristics.

At the end of the 19th century, cane fencing lost its sporting character and turned into a martial art. In 1899 a book by J. Charlemont was published, which stressed power and defense. He criticizes a number of classic strokes and concludes: "these strokes are useless for serious defense, because they are made with a half open hand. They are aimed toward the front with an almost straight arm, using only the power of the wrist or the hand; or from above toward the head, also from the wrist. It is very easy to understand that the cane has it full capacity, if it is hit with great strength, which is impossible if the fist is bent or extended and the wrist is moving. It is much more dangerous, for the attacker, to firmly hold the cane. The energy is increased by turning the shoulder, the arm, the lower arm, the wrist and the hand. The blows are also strong, when given from further away, and their power increases with the power of the muscle the further away they are. One can not imagine how bad such a blow can be. The bent arm, which is as much as possible pulled to the back, draws a speedy circle, and, if well aimed, hits the opponent, usually rendering him out of action, because in this movement, the combination of the lowering of the shoulder and the momentum of the arm and wrist, increase the speed and hence the power of the blow. This is the principle, one could almost say the secret, behind our classes."

The classical fencing techniques are described in "L'art de la canne," but only to improve the flexibility of the wrist and to hold the cane in a more natural position.

In 1901 the English magazine "Pearson's" published a two volume, 22 page illustrated series about "Self defense with a cane."

Stick fencing and self defense

Fig. 43 A "Brevet de Canne," a diploma, signed by witnesses, which confirmed the participation in a cane fencing tournament.

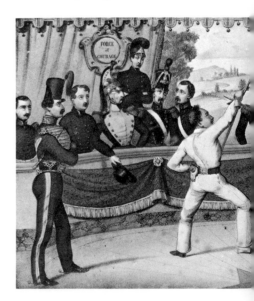

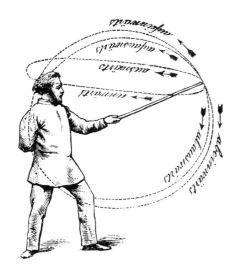

Fig. 44 The technique of circling the cane, as shown in Jacob Happel's "Geraethe Fechten," 1877.

The author E.W. Barton-Wright shows how to defend oneself during bad times against aggressors who come in large numbers or against an aggressor with a knife. Besides some fencing elements, his tools are very rough. He pulls the opponents leg with a crooked handle and makes him fall. He grabs him with the crook at the neck and pushed his head toward the ground, to hit his nose with the knee. He strikes the cane at ankles, knees and shin bones.

The aimed blows against the pain zones and nerve centers of the human bodies are the basis for the cane techniques by Bruce Tegner. In the United Stated he is an authority in self defense and has written two dozen books on the subject, among them two about battles with umbrellas and canes. In addition to the European cane fencing he also makes use of Asian martial arts techniques. The book was published in 1972.

In Munich I have met police officer Siegfried Lory, 6th Dan and instructor for modern self defense techniques, who includes a walking stick in his training programs. He uses a simple walking stick with a round handle and rubber ferrule, which turns into an extended arm with leverage effect, rather than a weapon. In combination with Jiu-Jitsu techniques, it is used systematic and effectively. The concept is that walking stick bearers are not helpless creatures using a walking aide. All they need to know is how to use the stick properly.

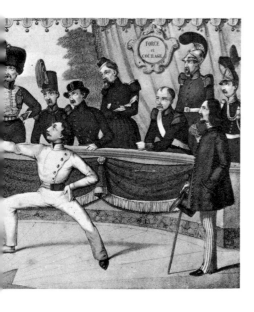

The cane industry started in the Biedermeier period

The commercial cane industry started at the transition from the 18th to the 19th century. The "trade prints," which were dedicated to a series of towns and their street vendors, also show cane sellers, as for example the man from Paris in 1760 who offers "good canes" and from a bundle of canes pulls one which is especially large. In Hamburg, Professor Christoph Suhr published a series of 120 prints in 1808, one of which is called "the town crier in Hamburg" and shows a man carrying suspenders in one hand and canes in the other and who cries "Walking sticks?"

The cane industry in Germany was founded during the Biedermeier (the Biedermeier style appears in 1815 and runs through 1848) and developed over the course of a few years according to the commission report of the German Industrial Fair in Munich 1854. The industry was not yet as important as the English cane industry, where one single manufacture would make up to half a million canes per year, or as the French one, which employed several thousand workers. In 1847 there were 165 cane manufacturers in Paris. Quote: "The German industry made a lot of progress over the last ten years, especially with respect to selling, which means that millions of Goulds, which used to be spent abroad, actually go to the national industry. The manufacture of canes is mainly done by turners. Several years back the German turner would not bother with cane production as it was considered an inferior trade; after seeing how much is to be made in this business from younger craftsmen who have returned from abroad, they now consider it as a good substitute for the crashed market in pipe production. With respect to elegance, the French industry is, as we have to admit openly, far superior."

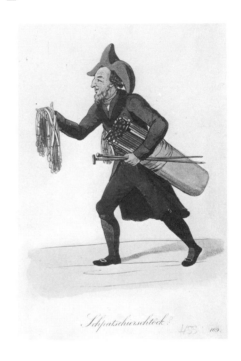

Fig. 45 Cane vendor, colored print by Ch. Suhr, 1808, from "Der Ausruf in Hamburg."

The "Stockmeier" Story

A typical example is the career of Heinrich Christian Meyer, who transformed himself from a carpenter to the largest cane manufacturer in Europe. His father Joachim had moved from the country to Hamburg at the moment the continental blockade brought unemployment. As a trained carpenter he started making walking sticks and sent his 8 year old son Heinrich Christian out, originally with a handful and later with an specially constructed cane chest, to the stock exchange building where he peddled the canes. A series about Hamburg shows the little "Canemeyer" in front of the Westermann stationary store. The name "Canemeyer" became permanent and in 1817 he founded the company H.C. Meyer, which manufactured canes, especially those covered with fish bone. He had learned how to work with fish bone from a special manufacturer in Bremen, who made rods for umbrellas and corsets out of fish bone. After a few years, a wood trading company was added, the carving of ivory for handles was added and in 1833 a steam engine was ordered from London. The steam engine was described as a "miracle, which turned into a tourist attraction in Hamburg." Around 1850 H.C.Meyer had between 200 and 300 employees and his cane factory was considered the biggest on earth. In addition, a trading company was started for mother of pearl, walrus tusks, hippopotamus teeth, horn, coconuts, tortoise and similar products used for handles and decorations. In 1856 a factory for the manufacture of hard rubber combs was added. Canes were also made from this material, which was considered a substitute for fish bone.

At the Industrial Fair in London in 1851 the company, now in the hands of the two sons of the old "Canemeyer" and his son-in-law F. Traun, showed the largest selection of canes: "no less than 500 different kinds." The Meyer colored lithograph catalogue of the same period lists the following materials for shafts: besides different woods, cane are made of hard rubber, some full some covered with wood; canes are made of fish bone, wood covered or braided and from full fish bone.

There were many types of handles: ivory dog and horse heads, hippopotamus tooth, antlers, olive wood, hazel wood, oak wood, brass and silver; tilted blossoms in ivory; lady's legs with boots in ivory and antler; horse legs also in the same material; heads of foxes, boars, cats, frogs made of various woods; flowers, leaves and bird's wings made of ivory; a bent finger of ivory; eagles and other bird's heads with large beaks (forming the handles) made of different materials, a monkey's head with a cap, which forms the handle, of two-tone horn, grotesque male heads made of antlers.

These male heads with long noses, the antler forming the over sized nose, were popular images on German walking sticks. They had their opposites in the militant nose men characters of Ch. Schmolze in the "Muenchner Bilderbogen," published since 1849.

An official document made reference to the figural handles: "... that even in large factories these handles were made by a small number of workers, usually 3 or 4, who, without any artistic training,

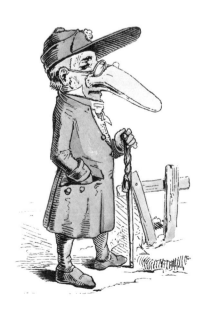

Fig. 46 This nose man from "Der Muenchner Bilderbogen" Nr. 18 is more peaceful than martial, circa 1850.

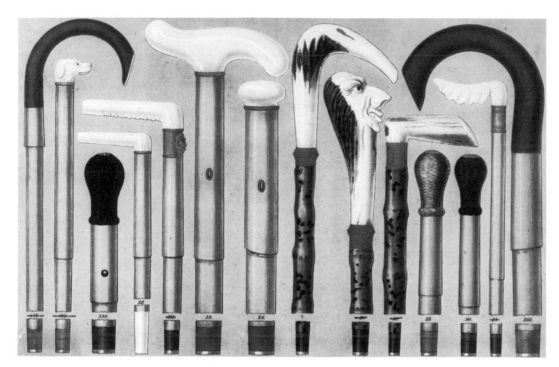

Fig. 47 Catalogue page from the H.C. Meyer Company, circa 1852. The shafts are either "Sugar cane," or "Tiger bamboo," as noted by hand. Hand colored.

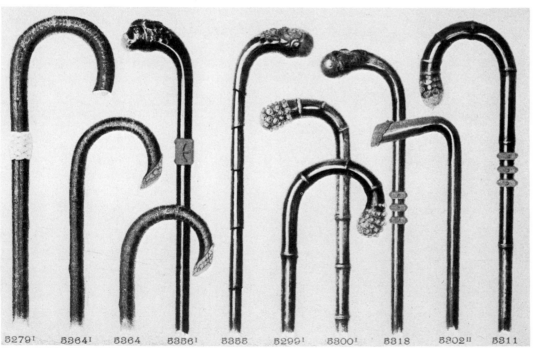

Fig. 48 Catalogue page of the same company, circa 1870. "Walking sicks with crooked handles and metal ferrules." Lithograph.

carved the forms of human beings and animals with specific impressions and characteristics with unbelievable truth and great taste."

Compared to this, the "Catalog for special canes by H.C. Meyer Jr. in Harburg/Elbe" twenty years later seemed boring. Besides a crocodile, a boar's head, a rabbit, and an Indian head, which are all elongated, made of ivory or hippopotamus teeth with almost straight handles, nothing figural is left. Handles are made of horn, with metal decoration. Straight handles with applied metal and crooks were also produced. The cane production is totally automated by now. Let us examine, how, at the turn of the century, canes were made. I would like to use the report of the commission of the German governments under the tariff union.

Visit to a cane factory around 1850

The commission had the opportunity to visit the facility of the Barnett Meyers Company in London, which currently manufactures 60,000 partridge canes, 80,000 bamboo canes, 110,000 malacca canes, 100,000 dragon canes (from the rotang palm family), 15,000 rattan and 144,000 canes made of oak, ash, apple thorn and maple wood. The unbelievable number of canes which were sold during that period is also stressed by the fact that the Chinese harbor of Canton shipped 1.2 million canes and bamboos every year. But come along to the warehouses of Barnett Meyers: "Indeed one wanders along rows of piles of woods and canes, which are stored to dry, usually for an extended period of time, one thinks one is in a fire wood storage, that is how plain these materials seem, which nevertheless are worth thousands of pounds. One is not amazed anymore when realizing that the most simple cane has to go through a workers hand at least 20 times before somehow reaching an acceptable form; more elaborate canes require an even higher number of steps."

First the bark is removed, which is done by boiling the cane for hours in order, for example, to avoid injuring the wart-like knots, which are so typical for apple wood. The softened bark can easily be removed with the fingers nails. Then the cane gets a crook at one end as handle: sticks or canes are covered with hot, moist sand, until the wood is soft and flexible and can be bent without breaking into the desired form, which remains when the wood is cold again. The art is to find the right temperatures for each individual type of wood. The straightening of the stick is done with dry sand heated on iron plates. After the stick turned hot like glowing iron, the stick is pulled in both directions along a groove which is cut into a piece of wood until it is absolutely straight. "Knots, bamboo rings and spiral turns are considered beautiful depending on the fashion. These forms are seldom found or are uneven in nature. They are frequently achieved by using graders and files."

After the sticks have been straightened and filed, the surface is polished with fish skins and sandpaper, colored and finally varnished and lacquered. Sometimes the canes are covered with printed patterns. This is more common on the continent, were manual labor is not as expensive as in England. Finally the different handles are attached.

The price of canes around 1854

I have found a price list for the C. Hedinger Company, which lists prices per dozen. The prices are in Goulds-Kreuzer currency, which in 1837 in the "Munich Convention" had the following values: 1 Gould = 60 Kreuzer, 1 Kreuzer = 4 Pfennig. The exchange rate to the Taler: 35 Gulden = 20 Taler, which is the 24 1/2 Gould rate, which until 1857 was valid between Northern and Southern Germany.

The average weekly salary of a worker at 14 hours a day and 6 days a week was 3 Goulds.

"Walking sticks,
laurier or partridge canes...   *9 Goulds 36 Kreuser to 12 goulds*

Walking canes, local black-, white thorn,
vines, palms; bamboos and pepper cane,
manila and malacca cane...   *4 goulds to 60 goulds*

Rhinoceros horn canes per piece...   *11 goulds"*

Mr. Thonet and Mr. Dangerfield make an invention

How the handles were bent by hand was seen at the Meyer Company in London. About 30 years later it was done by machine. William Dangerfield from Chalford in Gloucestershire got a mechanical bending machine patented in 1864.

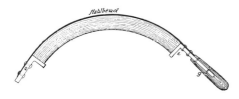

Fig. 49 A so called iron planchet (band), which keeps the handle from breaking during the bending process.

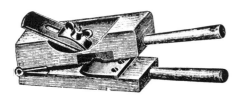

Fig. 50 Flap plane which brings the shaft, after it has been rounded with the plane, into a conical form.

Fig. 51 The circular grader rotates on the turning lathe, smoothing the forms and rough surfaces. This work requires lots of experience.

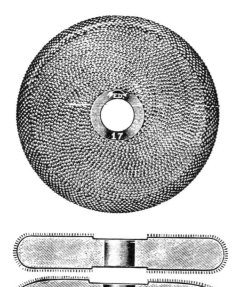

In 1832 the furniture maker Michael Thonet in Boppard/Rhinehad invented a method for bending glued veneer with hot glue in molds into any shape. He mainly used the technique for the backs of his chairs, which, as with Viennese coffee house tables, are still made today. Thonet chairs are by far the most appealing and comfortable chairs of this kind. The bending of wood was always difficult and had a high rate of breakage. The bending requires experience and knowledge and requires wood of specific kinds and qualities.

The bending technique was very important for the new industry, because it saved lots of wood compared to cutting a curved wooden shape from a flat piece. Bent wood becomes stronger too, the proper treatment means that the wood is not stretched outside and compressed inside. This is achieved by bandaging the softened wood, then bending steel holds the wood in such a way that it can not stretch on the outside. The resultant bending is achieved solely by compressing the fibers of the inner curve. This is the idea behind the invention by Mister Dangerfield, which in an article in "Camber's Journal" from February 11, 1871 is described as follows: "the camber now can fulfill the miracle of bending a stick, as if it were iron wire, without it breaking or bouncing back. The wood is soaked for an extended period of time in wet sand in order not to break it. A flexible metal band is attached to the outer curve of the bend, then the upper end is set into a metal mold, which will determine the diameter of the bend. The other end of the stick is turned until it points in the opposite direction. During this process the metal band puts more and more pressure against the extending wood fibers, hindering them from either breaking or rupturing. After the handle has reached its bend the process has to be stopped, and the stick must be prevented from returning to its original form. Originally the cane was just left to cool to keep its form. The newest technique is to turn the handle over a gas burner."

These techniques were very sophisticated and, besides minor improvements, the cane industry had no further changes. Until its end in the 1930s — there are only a very small number or companies left — the industry always kept something of this bending craft.

Illustrations

In reference to the illustrations:
The provenance, age and meaning of the image quite often can
not determined with certainty, and therefore the word "probably"
is used in the descriptions of the illustrations, or the description
is omitted, if too much speculation would be necessary. The author is asking the readers who know more about such a piece to
share their knowledge with the author. Sizes are only given if the
image would be misleading otherwise. A normal handle is 9 to 12
cm long, a knob about 6 cm high.

Abbreviations:
H. = Half
C. = Century
H. = Height
L. = Length
D. = Diameter

1 *Bourgeois family. The mother is carrying a naked child on her arm, the father is wearing a fashionable wig and holding a cane with a golden knob. A little pug is sitting at their feet. The group is carved in ivory, with eyes set in ruby. The knob is in a gold acanthus leave setting on a malacca cane. Probably Dutch, 18th C., height of cane 100 cm. Sold at auction by Sotheby's Parke Bernet Monaco on May 25, 1975.*

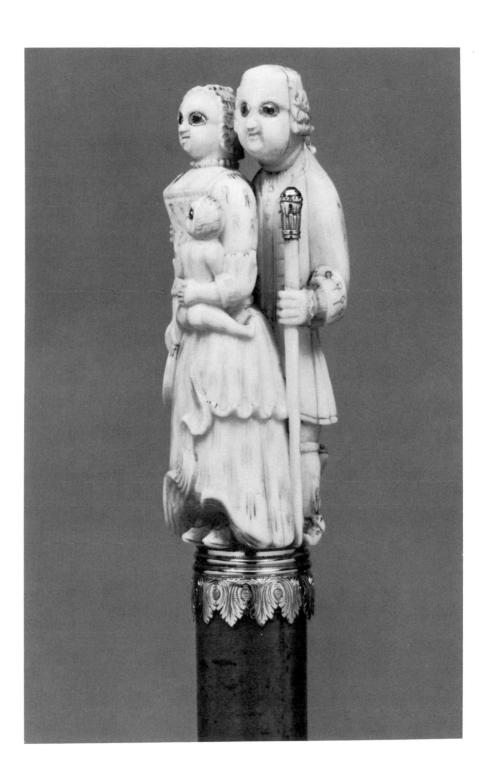

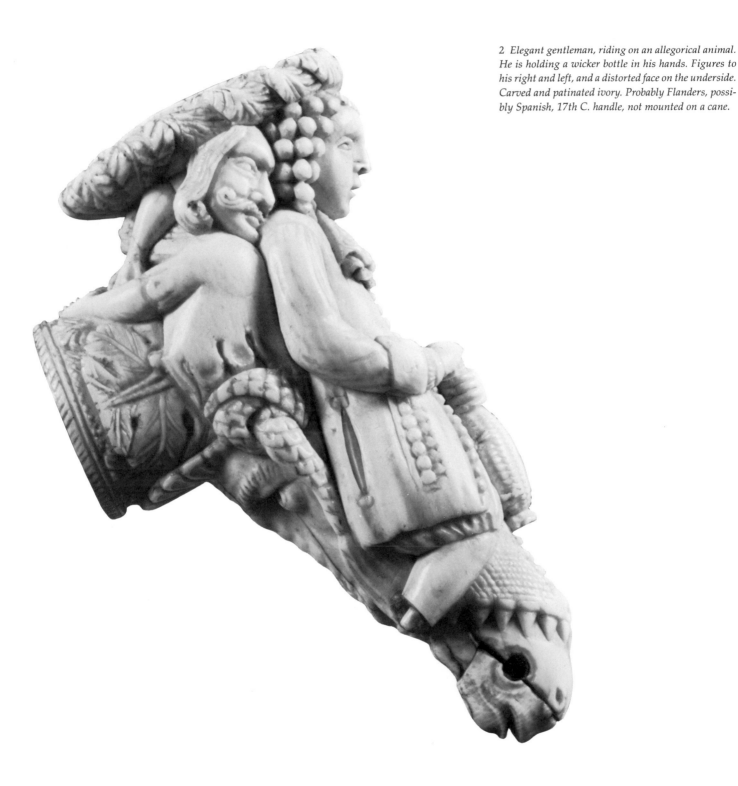

2 *Elegant gentleman, riding on an allegorical animal. He is holding a wicker bottle in his hands. Figures to his right and left, and a distorted face on the underside. Carved and patinated ivory. Probably Flanders, possibly Spanish, 17th C. handle, not mounted on a cane.*

3 Naked lady with dog. Reclining on pillows and a bed of leaves. Ivory with hairlines caused by age. The work of a Napoleonic prisoner of war (?), but probably earlier.

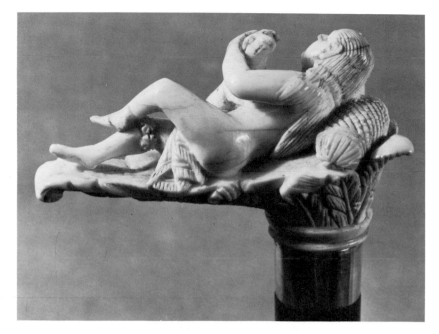

4 Allegorical image of a naked woman, tied to a ram. Ivory, carved in the round, with patina caused by age. The laterally engraved inscription "Andromede" refers to the Andromeda tale: The daughter of Kassiopeia should have been sacrificed to a beast, after having offended the Nereids. She was chained to a rock, but later freed by Perseus. Early French work, probably 16th C.

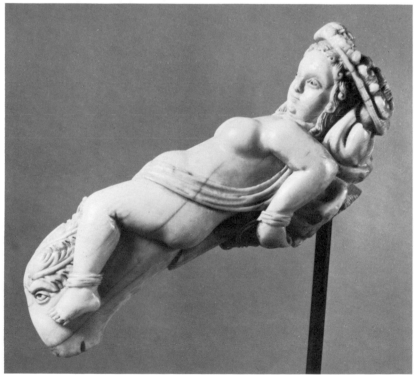

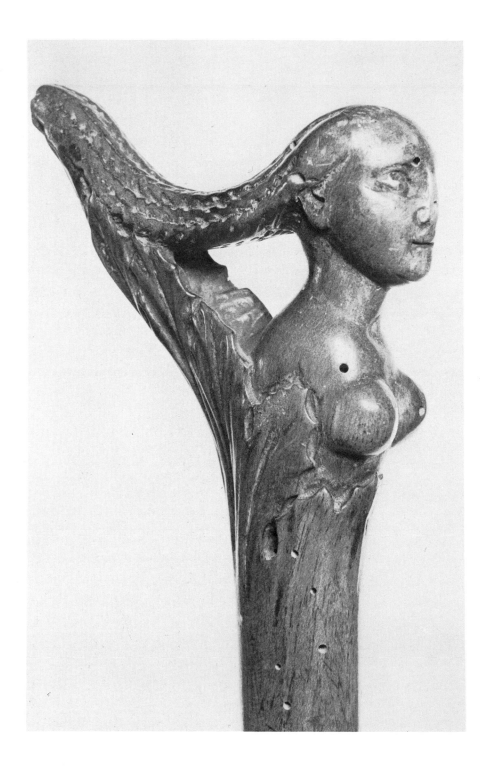

5 Female bust, emerging from an opening leaf calyx. The hair being the handle. Hard wood cane, carved from one piece. Face and bosom show wear. The ferrule: a hand made nail, drilled into the shaft. 18th C., L. 10 cm.

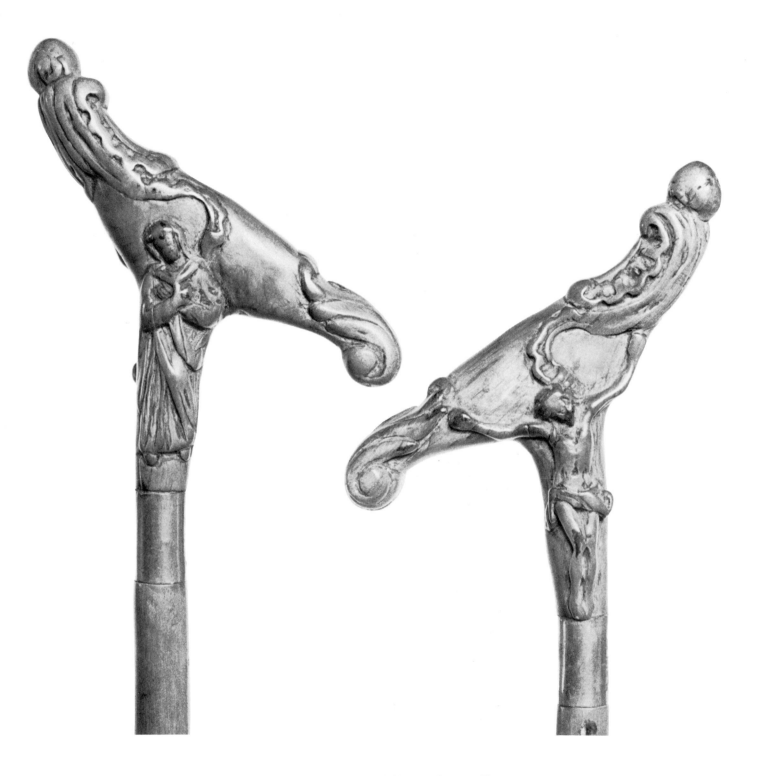

6, 7 *The grieving Mary and Christ on the cross. The handle is carved on both sides, ending in a very worn angels head with shell and scrolls. Fruitwood handle, bleached from hand sweat. The shaft is made from hazel nut wood, attached by a brass ring. Probably from the circle of the carver Joseph Teutschmann, Passau, 18th C. handle, L. 16 cm, wrought iron ferrule 15 cm long.*

8   *The ornaments, dates and names on these ivory knobs are applied with silver nails. This technique is called pique. From the left: "Lavrance Lugg" 1667; "D.T. 95" 1695, circa 1690. One iron and one silver ring. Both sold at Christie's London on December 12, 1977.*

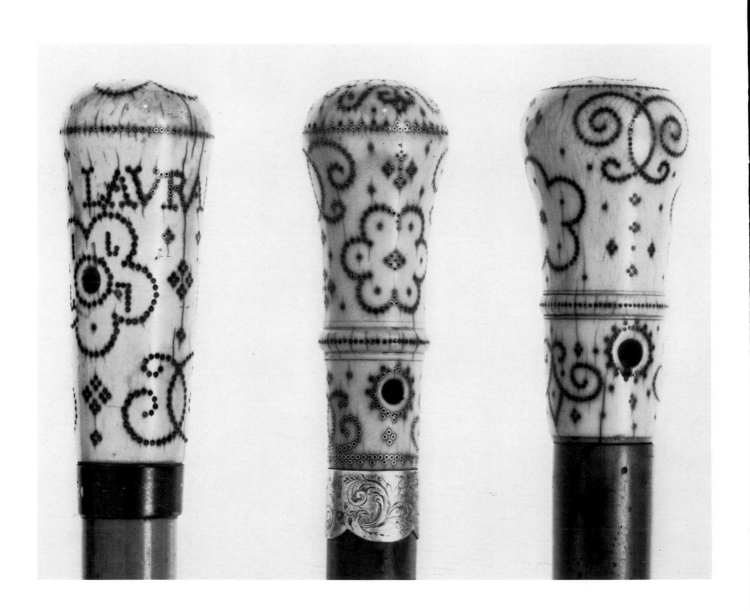

9 Pique on rhinoceros horn, English, circa 1700. Silver ring on malacca cane. Knob H. 11 cm.

10 Pique on ivory, English, circa 1730. Malacca cane, the knob has a star form decoration around the band hole. Height of knob 10 cm.

11 French Lady's cane painted with bows, quivers, shields and bands, Louis XVI period. Height of cane 130 cm.

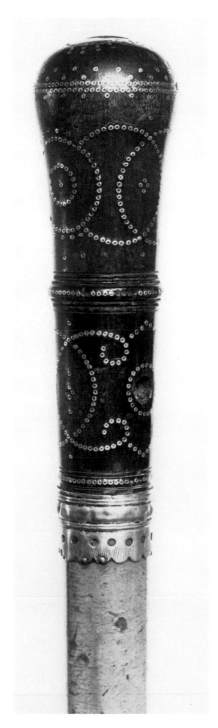

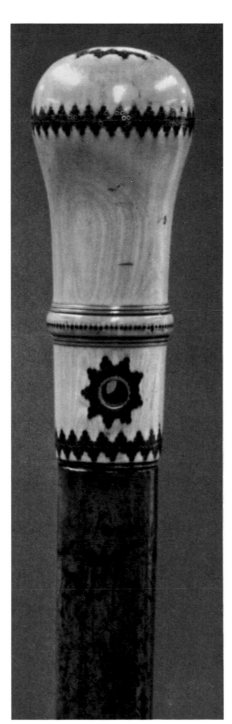

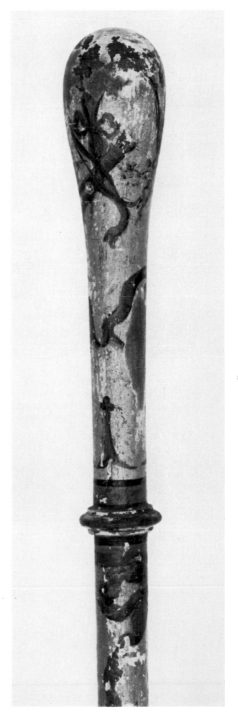

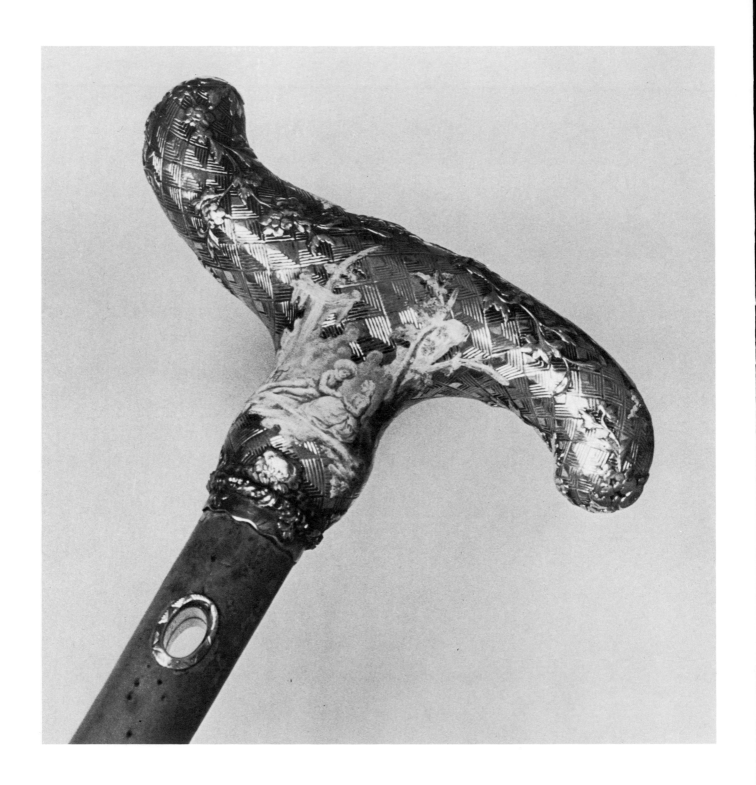

12 Cane with gold Fritz handle formerly belonging to
Frederick the Great. Rose gold with applied leaves,
enamel scenes in Delft blue/white. Malacca cane.
Hechingen/Baden-Wuerttemberg, Treasury of the
Hohenzollern castle.

13 Cylinder form knob in two-tone gold, decorated with green, white and blue enamel. Knob rings decorated with acanthus in low relief. Malacca cane. Paris, circa 1840.

14 Large presentation cane with turned silver knob, ebony shaft. France, end of the 18th C. Height of cane 118 cm. Previously in the collection of Sacha Guitry, sold on February 15, 1983 by Sotheby's Parke Bernet Monaco.

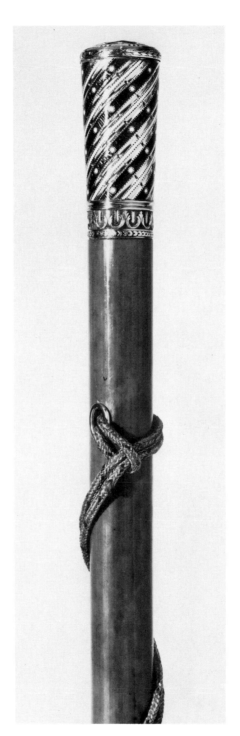

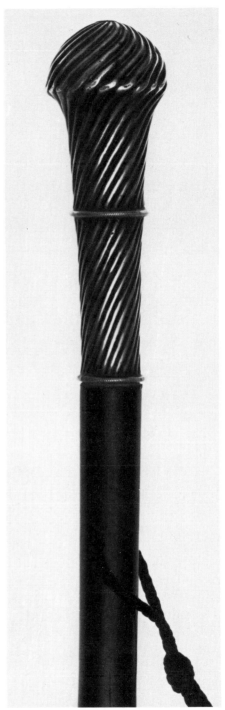

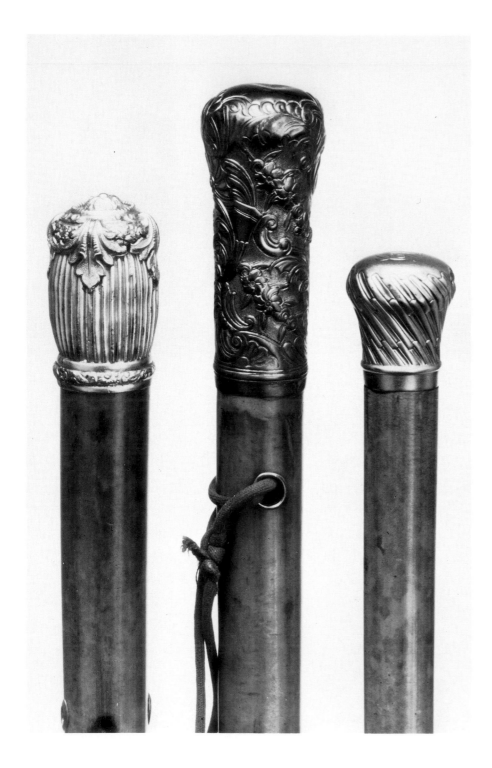

15 From the left: Gilded knob with acanthus leaf decoration on malacca cane. Probably English, middle 19th century, Height of knob 5.5 cm. — Gilded knob embossed with flowers and architectural rococo motifs on lone malacca cane with gold edged hole for the band, which was wrapped around the wrist of the bearer. Circa 1760. Height of knob 7.5 cm. Gold knob with bar form decoration and the initials "CND" on a malacca cane. Circa 1770. Height of knob 4 cm.

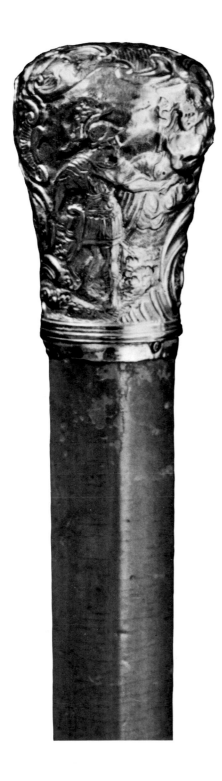
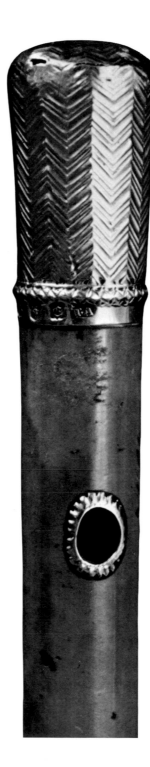
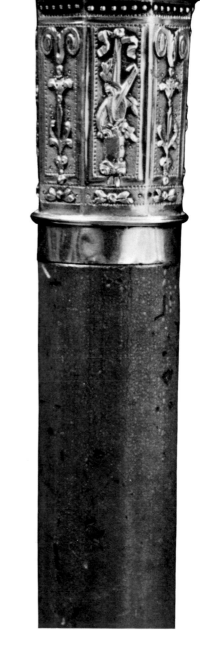

16 Massive gold knob, chased and engraved with mythological scenes and rocailles. Reddish malacca cane of the period. Probably French. Height of knob 4.5 cm.

17 Massive gold knob, hand chased, with herring bone pattern. Light malacca cane, gold edged hole. English hallmarks. Early 19th century, Height of knob 4.5 cm.

18 Tri color gold knob, octagonal, decorated with musical instruments. Malacca cane. High quality French craftsmanship, 18th Century. Height 5 cm.

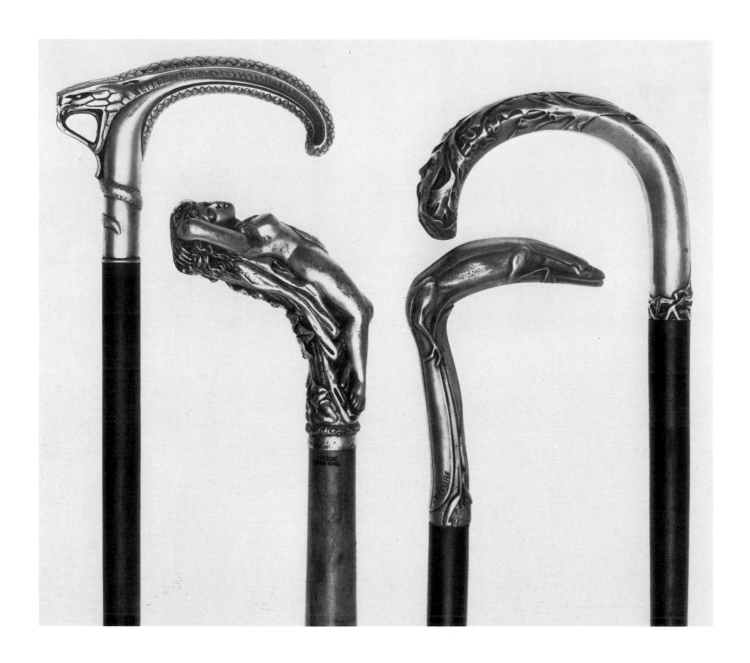

19 *From the left: Silver cobra head on an ebony shaft. Reclining nude, sil-*
vered, mounted on a malacca cane, signed Antoine, Palais Royal. — Sala-
mander in metal by de Feure on snake wood shaft — silver round handle with
floral decoration and a female head in the style of Mucha, snake wood.

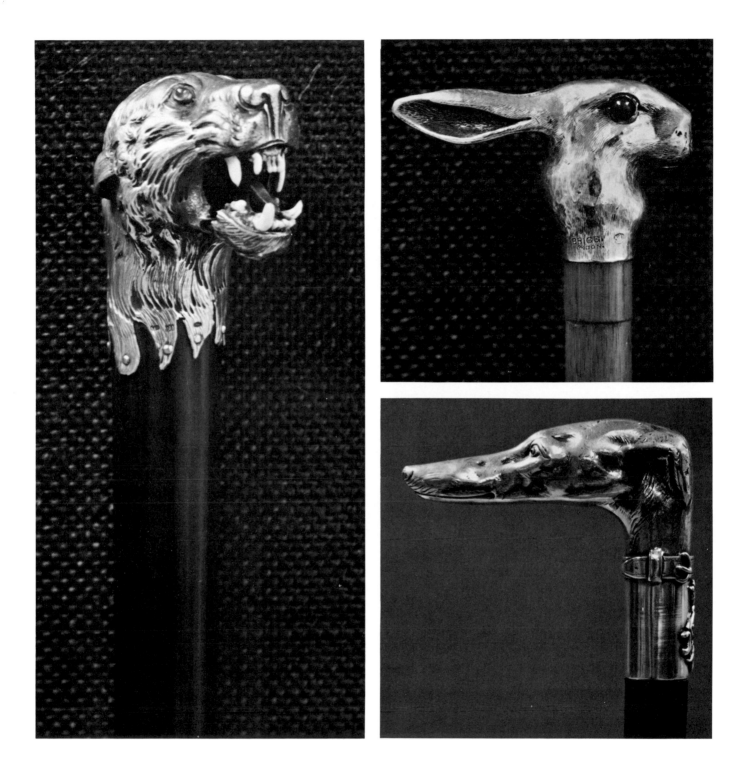

20-22 *Silver lion with movable chin and marten teeth. — hand chased rabbit head in silver from Brigg in London from circa 1912. Length 12 cm. — head of a greyhound, massive silver with finely chased surface. Raised monogram "S.J." and five pointed crown. Vienna, early 20th Century, Length 11 cm.*

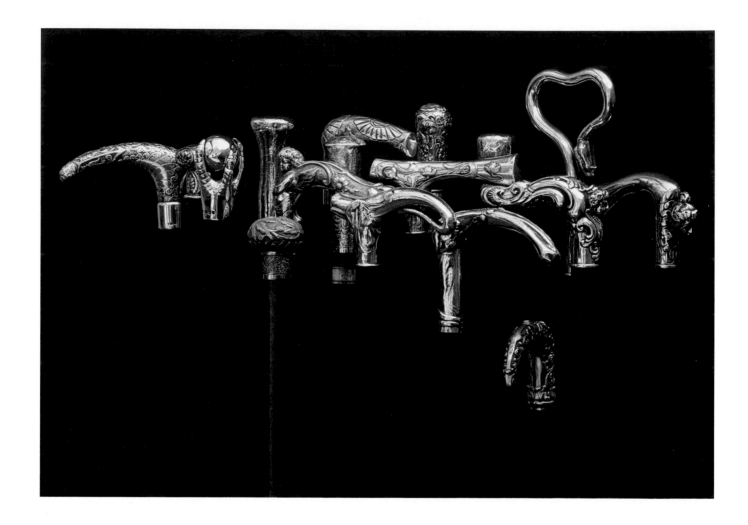

23   Embossed and molded silvered knobs from the Gruenderzeit (late 19th
Century) and the Jugendstil (early 20th Century). The lady's head on the right
in the style of Alphonse Mucha. French, German and English pieces. As a
reference to their size: The handle with the curved snake is 15 cm high overall.

24 Male head with fool's hat, Meissen number 269, Johann Christoph Ludwig Luecke, 1728. Silver collar as ring. Length 9.5 cm. Time of manufacture not available.

25 Court fool Joseph Froehlich, who was a model for Kaendler many times, is shown here as a rare cane handle. Meissen, 1743, Length 13.5 cm. Sold at auction by Sotheby's London on May 25, 1982.

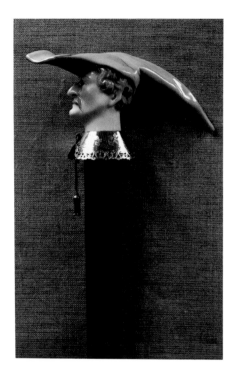

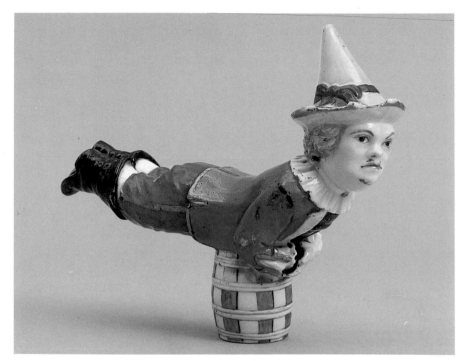

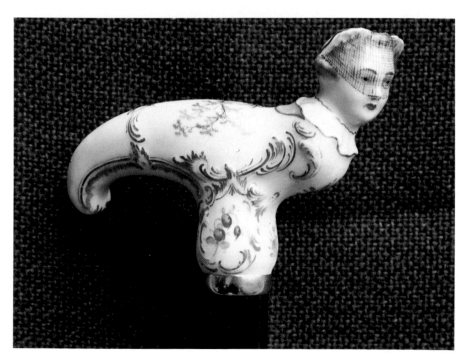

26 Female head with veil, a favorite subject for porcelain manufacturers. The handle back shows a painted landscape with a town in the background. Recent mounting on ebony wood cane. Probably 19th century. Length 12 cm.

27, 28 *Male head by Franz Anton Bustelli of the "Porcelain Manufacture Nymphengurg." In old archives it is listed as "Cane knob with boy's head." Still sold as Cork head without pint.*

29 *Blue porcelain ball for a knob with white applied foliate decoration and Eros on the top. English, Wedgwood, turn of the century. Height of knob 5.5 cm.*

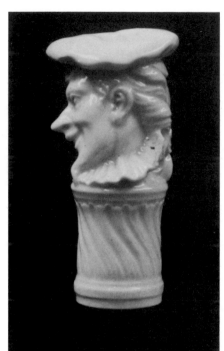

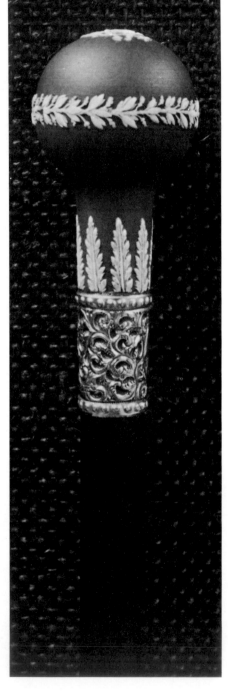

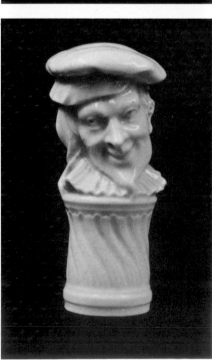

30 *This cylindrical French knob is decorated with pansies. Probably around 1770.*

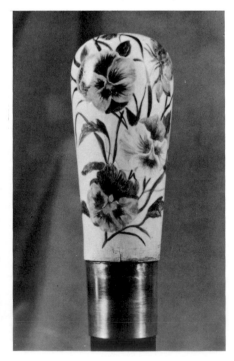

31 Head of a pug by Kaendler, yellow background with painted landscape. The handle
was converted into a seal. Meissen, 18th Century. Sold at Christie's London in October
1976.

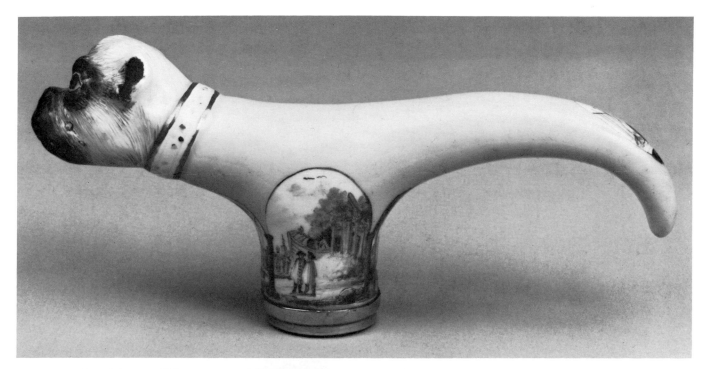

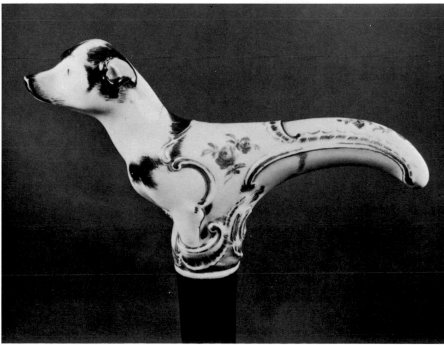

32 Hunting dog with floral decoration.
Maker unknown, possibly Chelse. 18th Century, Length 7.5 cm.

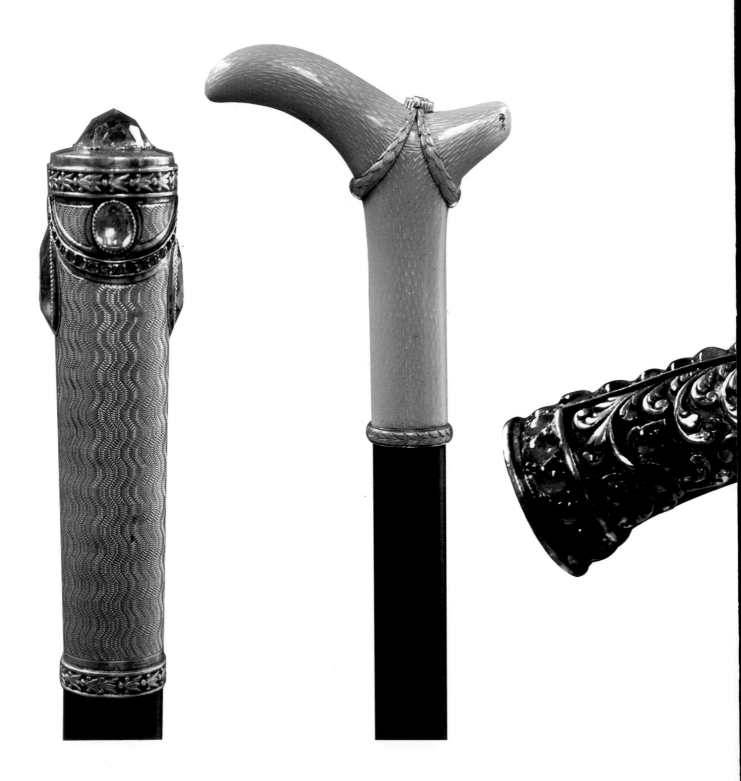

33 Handle with translucent enamel over engine turning. The knob is decorated with 5 yellow topaz. French (possibly Houillon), turn of the century (?), Height 8.5 cm.

34 Handle, translucent blue enamel over floral garlands and guilloched metal by Henrik Wigstoem from the shop of Carl Fabergé. Petersburg, circa 1900. Height 6.5 cm.

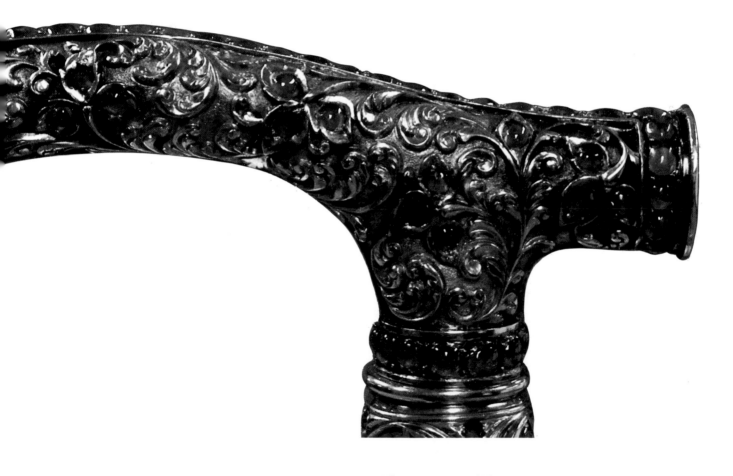

35 Fine heavy gold handle, chased and engraved with rocailles. The surface is set with
Burmese cabochon rubies. Screwed on handle
with compartment (for poison). India, 19th
century handle. Length 9 cm.

36   *Magnificent ivory knob with Baccarat style engraved decoration. Classical regency work, shaft in Guajuvira Palisander wood. English 19th Century. Height 7.5 cm.*

37   *The handle is curved to the outside for a right handed person, therefore it is very well positioned in the hand. Slim malacca case. Probably German.*

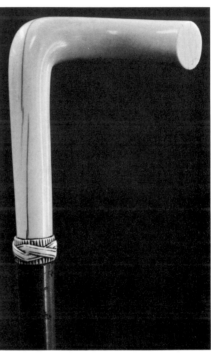

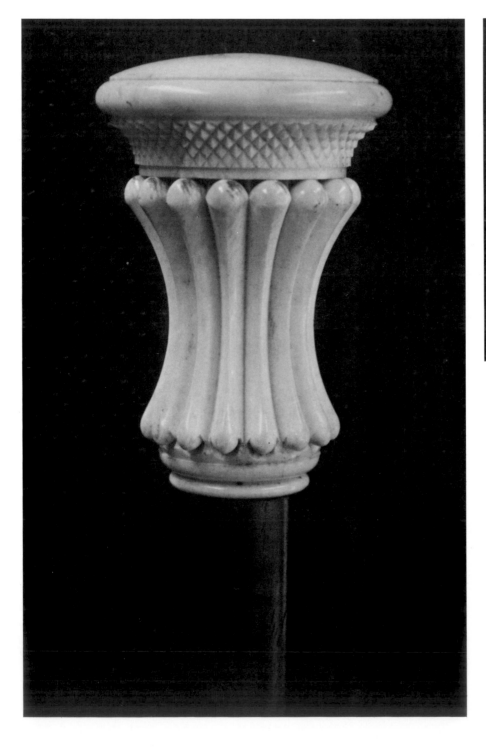

38 A fully sculptured woman is standing in a floral pattern cage, carved from one piece. Originally an Indian dagger, later converted into a cane, mounted on Palisander. 19th Century, Height 13.5 cm.

39, 40 Hand with key, carved in relief, the floral ornaments are engraved and stained in black with pigment or wax. Patina caused by age. Height 11.5 cm.

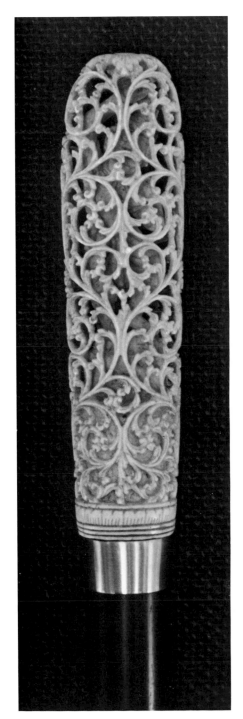

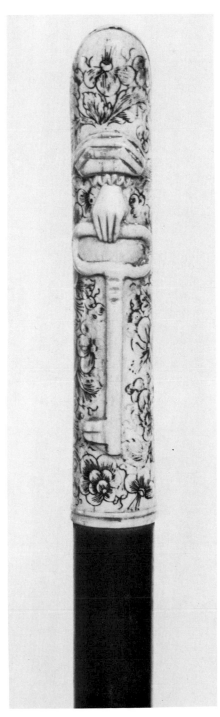

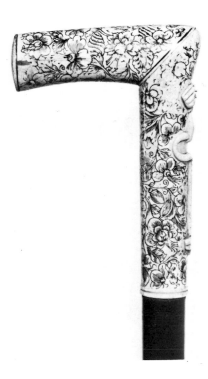

41 A satyr works as a barrel maker, while a naked woman is sitting in the barrel. Extraordinary craftsmanship on this cane with stylized trees and many putti. Masterpiece (?). End of 17th Century (?). Overall length 80 cm.

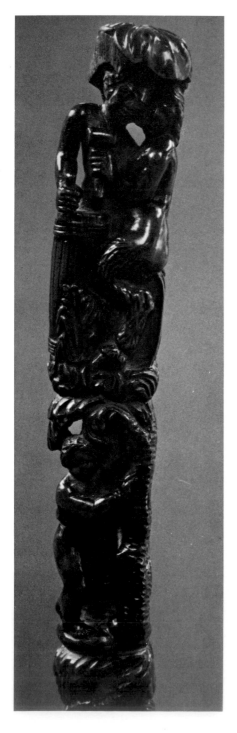

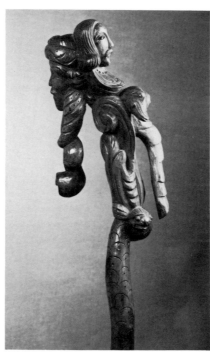

42 The root dictates the arrangement of heads and animals. Shaft and handle all of one piece, very finely carved. Probably 18th century.

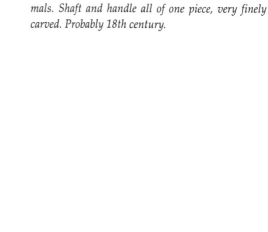

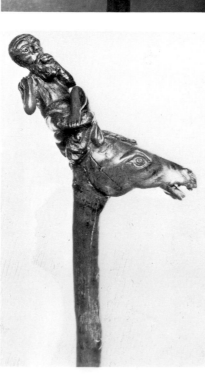

43 A finely carved old, naked man is sitting on the just as finely carved head of a horse, while holding his beard. Shaft and handle carved from one piece of very hard and thin wood. Probably 17th Century. Length of the horse's head 7 cm.

44 A root with three twigs is braided into a cane, the end piece carved as a man's bust, height 8 cm, simple carving and coloring.

45 Well carved animal's heads from one root. The whole cane made from one piece with hole for a band. Early piece.

46 Partial view of a farmer's cane carved from top to bottom (see also page 8). Primitive, diligent work. Age and provenance unknown.

47 Finely engraved cane with scenes from a fox hunt, the crest of the House of Hannover and a cricket scene. Detailed naive work from Victorian England.

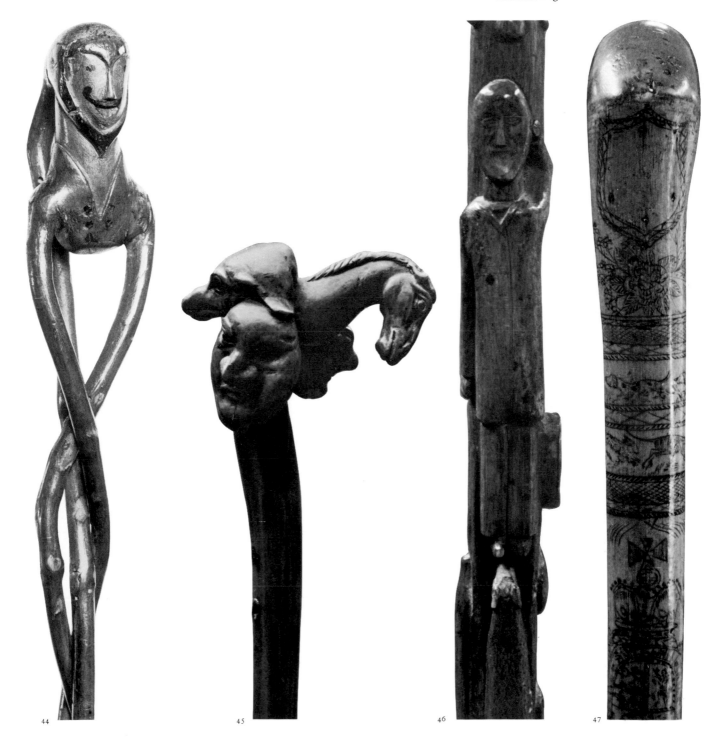

44   45   46   47

48 Grotesque portrayal of a Southern Black with monocle, sitting on a chair. Hard wood, carved, colored, realistic eyes and bone teeth. This subject is known in several variations, yet each cane is unique. Height 12 cm.

49, 50 Shepherd's cane with dolphin from Crete. The handle called "heri" is used to catch the sheep by its ankle. Illustration Nr. 49 was made and purchased in Crete in 197. Illustration Nr. 50 is made of a vine and is over 100 years old.

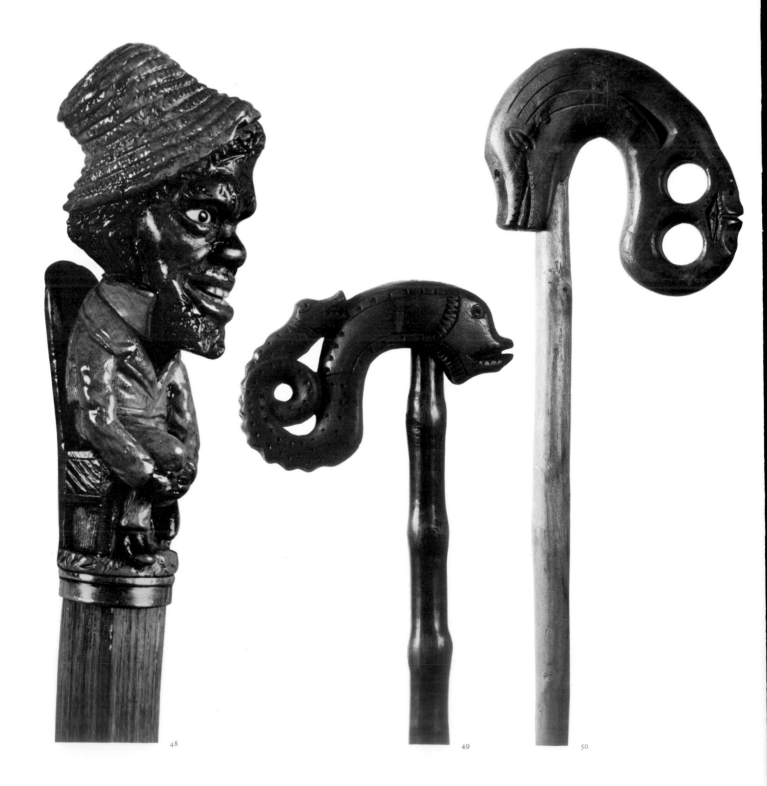

48

49

50

51 *Serpent, fish and horse's head are intertwined following the nature of the root. Provenance unknown.*

52 *Monkey's head with bone inlay, very finely carved and patinated. Either a seaman's or prisoner's work (?), early 19th Century.*

53 *A dragon-crocodile creature with a ball in its mouth is the handle of this cane which is carved out of one piece of blackthorn. 19th Century, Length 16.5 cm.*

54 *An entanglement of forest animals and plants is carved all over this cane, the knots are deer and bear's heads. Snakes are forming the handle ending in a lizard. Soft wood. Probably alpine.*

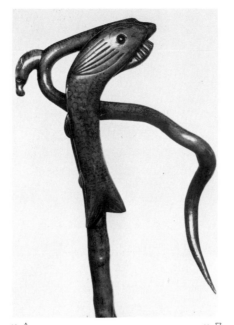

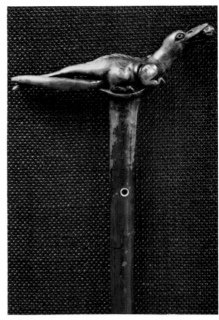

51 △   52 ▽   53 △   54 ▽

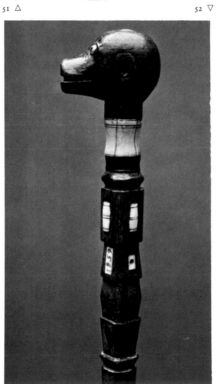

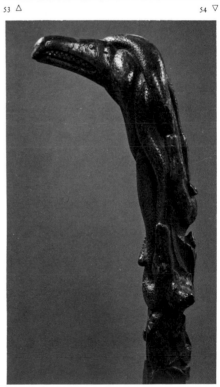

55 *This plain German hiking cane is made of chestnut wood and set with "cane nails." "Cane nails" are small plaques or figures in metal or, nowadays, plastic which can be bought at tourist attractions and applied to the hiking cane. A tradition started after the Second World War.*

56 *Water snakes and eels are depicted on fishermen's canes from China. Carved from ferrule to handle in one curved piece.*

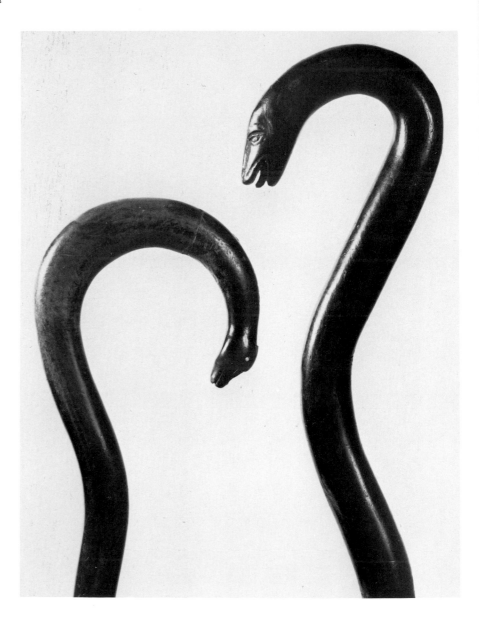

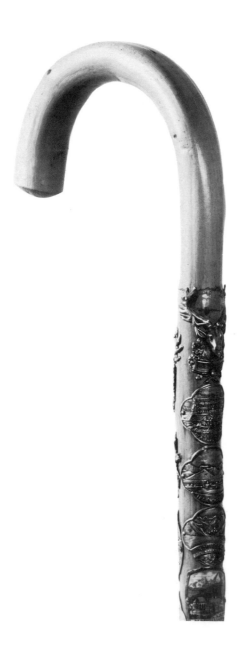

57 Left: Shepherd's staff taller than a man, from northern France. Right: Scottish Shepherd's staff with horn
handle in "neck crook" form, which were used to catch
sheep at their neck.

58 Old handle type "raven's beak" = bec de corbin was
rarely used as a working staff despite its useful form.
This staff contains a dagger.

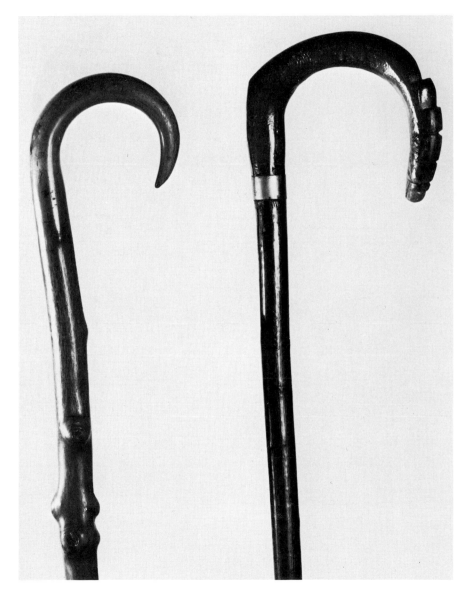

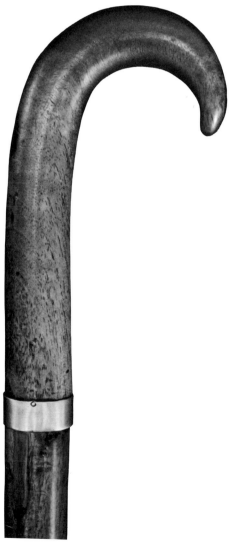

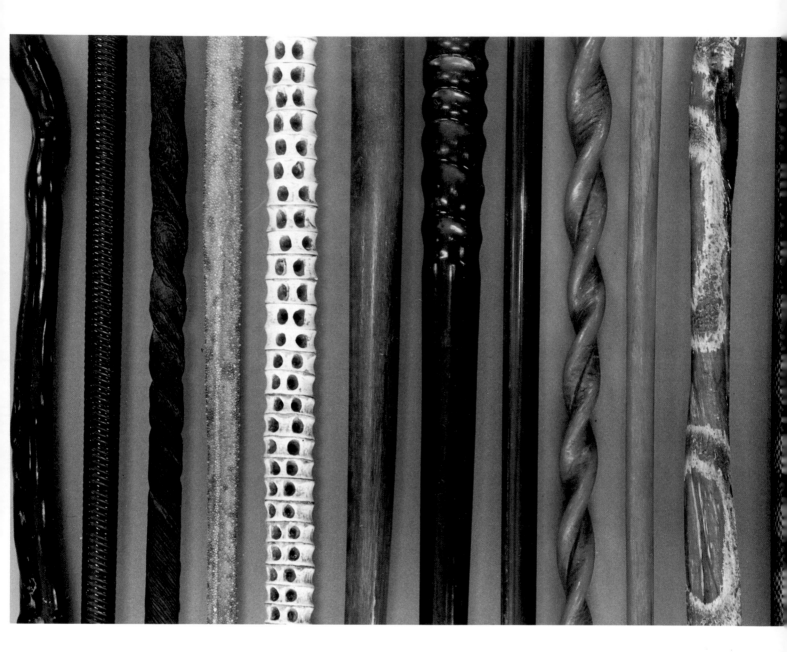

59 *From left to right: Black coral (horn coral); polished fish bone; unpolished fish bone; sting of a ray; back bone of a killer shark; rhino horn; horn of the African antelope; horn shaft; turned steer haunch without metal core; steer haunch on metal core; Texan steer haunch with fire marks on metal core, snake skin.*

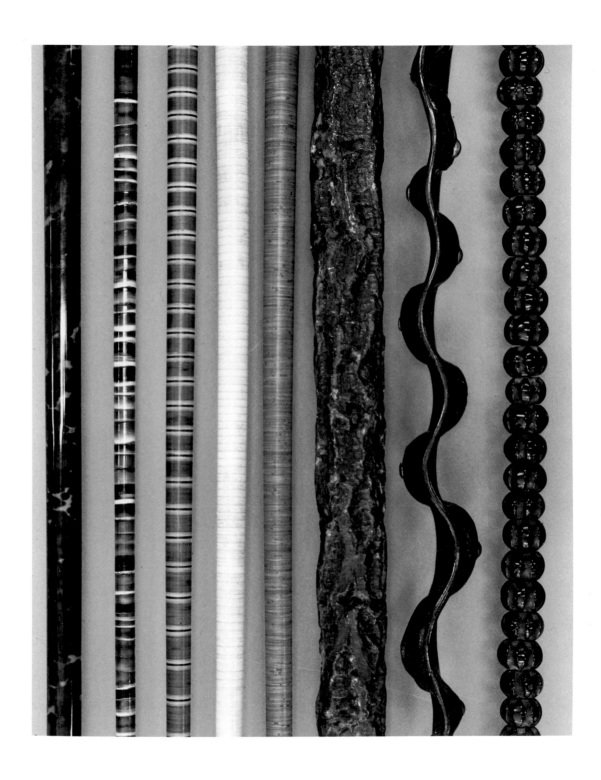

60 From left to right: Tortoise shell, horn discs, leather discs, paper discs, cork discs, all on metal cores; cork tree; tropical gigantic bean trees, decorated with nails; tropical cores and nuts on metal core.

61 *Antlers with rosette, used as handle of a hunter's cane. Exceptional Length 23 cm.*

62 *Horn of a chamois buck and an antelope are used as handles on these walking canes from the turn of the twentieth century. The one on the left is engraved with the names of Swiss spas.*

63 *A ram's horn with double winding, typical for Dorset sheep, Scotland, 20th Century.*

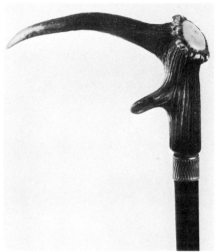

61 △

62 ▽

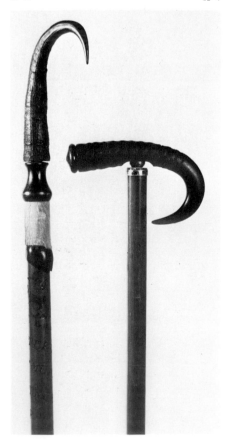

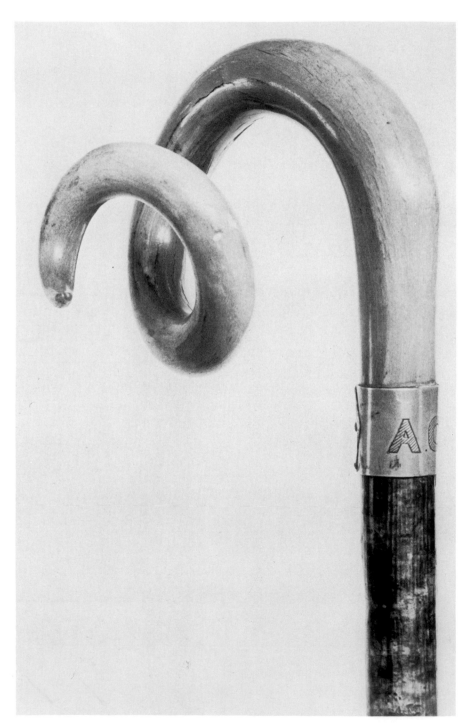

64 *A cane braided in straw from Burgenland (Austria).*

65 *This cane is covered with the skin of a sting ray or a shark.*

66 *Pitch covered rope braided into sophisticated patterns and knots. Typical seaman's work from the period of sailing vessels. Diameter of knob (= turkish knob) 7 cm.*

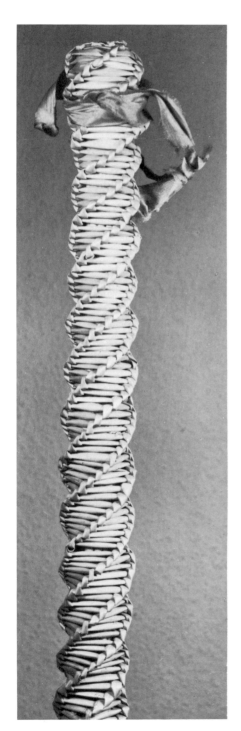

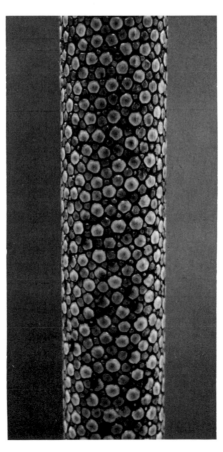

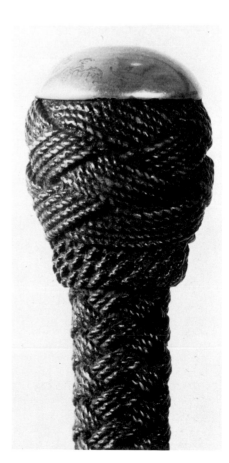

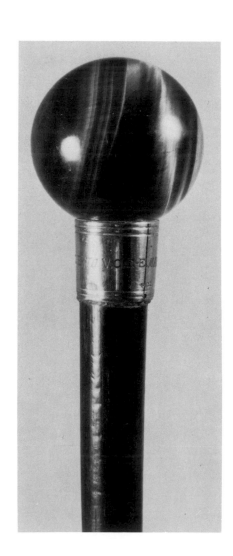

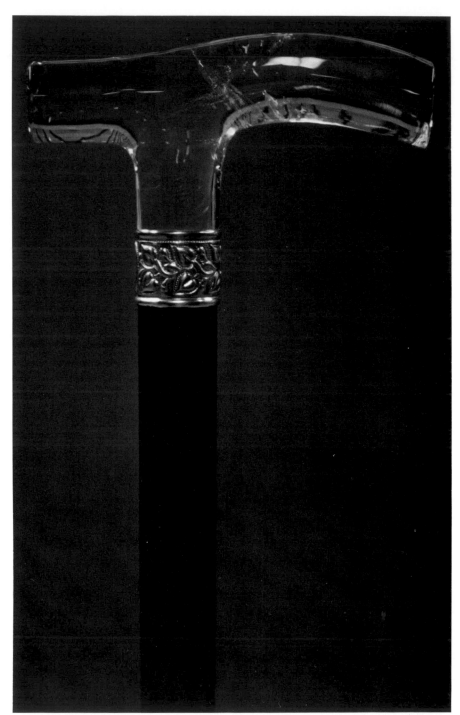

67 Ball form tiger's eye knob. Diameter 5 cm.

*68 Large crystal handle. Probably Russian, around the
turn of the twentieth century. Length 11 cm.*

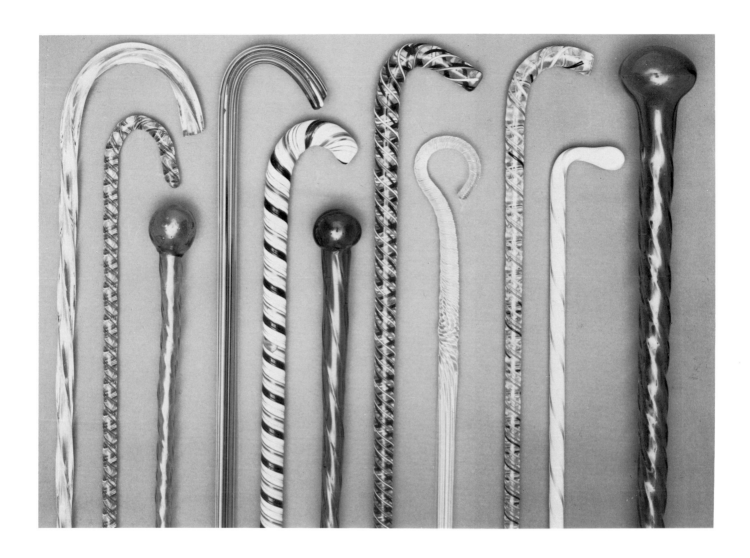

69 Glass canes for recruits in various techniques and sizes. In clear or poly-
chrome glass, hollow or solid shaft, in spiral form, or with applied color threads.
Normandy, circa 1850. Overall height between 83.5 cm and 119 cm. These
canes from the collection of Andre Luguet were sold by Sotheby's Parke Bernet
Monaco as one lot with 21 pieces.

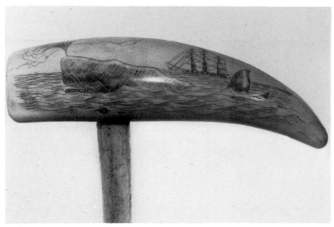

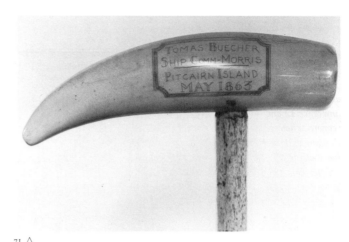

70 △

71 △

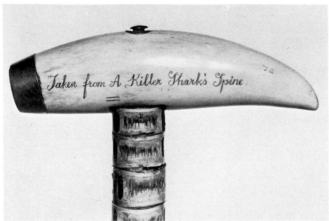

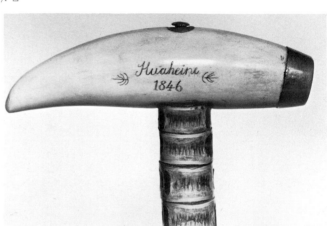

72 △   74 ▽   73 △   75 ▽

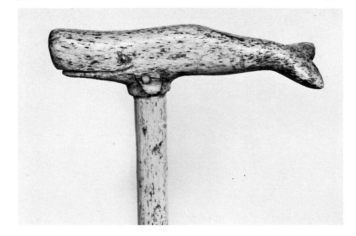

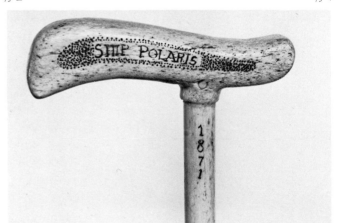

70, 71 Whale tooth with scrimshaw of a whaling scene, inscribed on the back and dated. Shaft made from whale bone. 1863, Length 16.5 cm

72, 73 Whale tooth, set in silver. Inscribed and dated. Mounted on the spine of a killer shark. 1846. Length 15 cm.

74 Carved whale with gold nails as eyes, carved from a whale bone and ivory mount. Length 13 cm.

75 Whale bone handle, inscribed and dated. The "Polaris" had been caught in ice in 1871. Length 13 cm.

76 From left to right: Well patinated, spiral carved whale bone shaft with handle made from a hippopotamus tooth inlaid with tortoise. Overall height 104 cm. — Sharks spine with silver knob, London hallmark from 1856. Very flexible. — Turned and hollowed whale bone shaft with tortoise decoration and sea lion tooth knob. — Heavy, unfinished Narwhal tooth with wooden knob, Circumference 12 cm. — Turned narwhal tooth with silver covered knob and ring, silver set ring for hole. — Shark's spine with ivory ball. — Large slightly treated narwhal tooth with handle made from hippopotamus tooth, silver bell form ring. Liverpool 1892. Overall Height 98 cm. — Bleached whale bone, turned in the upper section, but made from one piece.

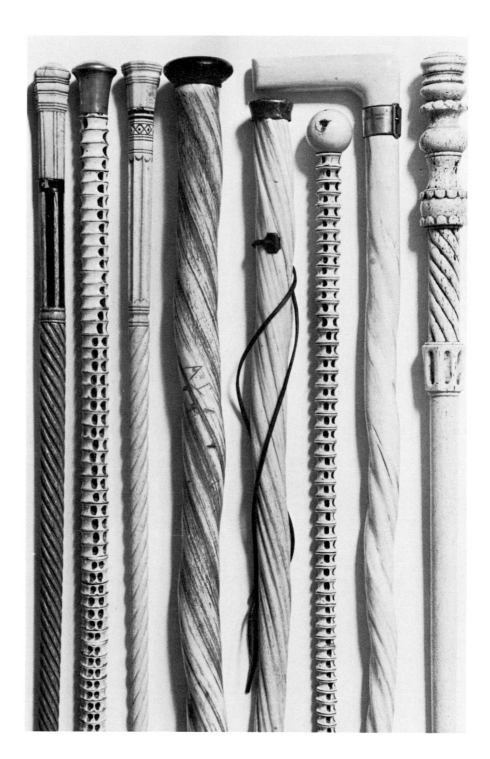

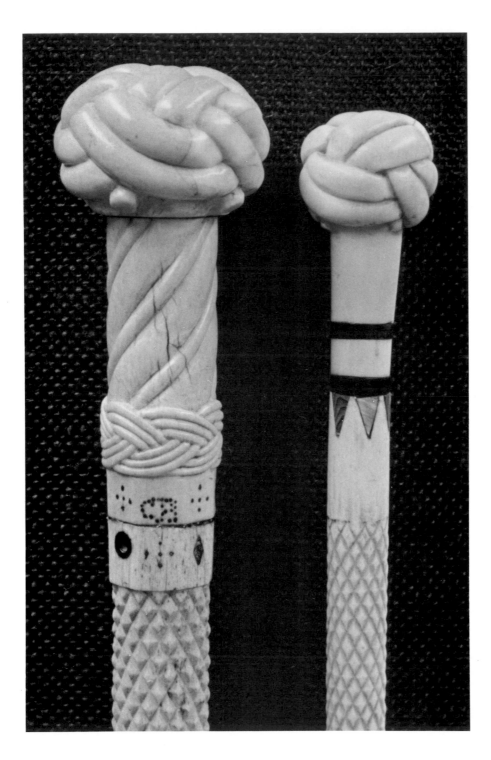

77 Handles carved from sperm whale tooth in the form of a Turkish knot are quite common among the whale bone canes. From the two illustrated examples, the one on the right is in usual size, emphasizing the extraordinary size of the one on the left. The inlays are in silver on the left and in mother of pearl and black wood on the right.

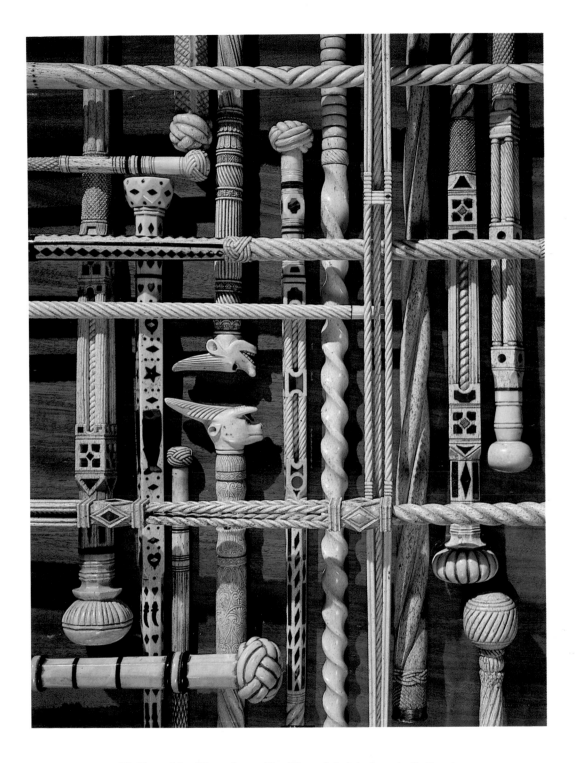

78 The variety of the craftsmanship of these whaler's is shown in the French collection in this illustration, very rare and fragile filigree canes, the two heads in the middle are rare and mystic. The different materials and the different porosity of those materials can be well distinguished.

79 Head of an Indian chief with head feathers in silver, is very decorative, probably American but not Native American. Probably first third of the 20th Century.

80 The squatting man with cap, which, only a European would see as a penis symbol, is from Bali. Behind his back is a beast, probably Garuda, the celestial bird. Horn carving, 20th Century, Height 10 cm.

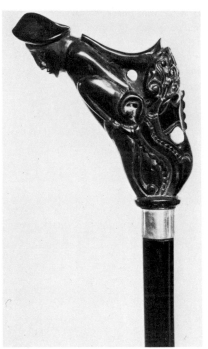

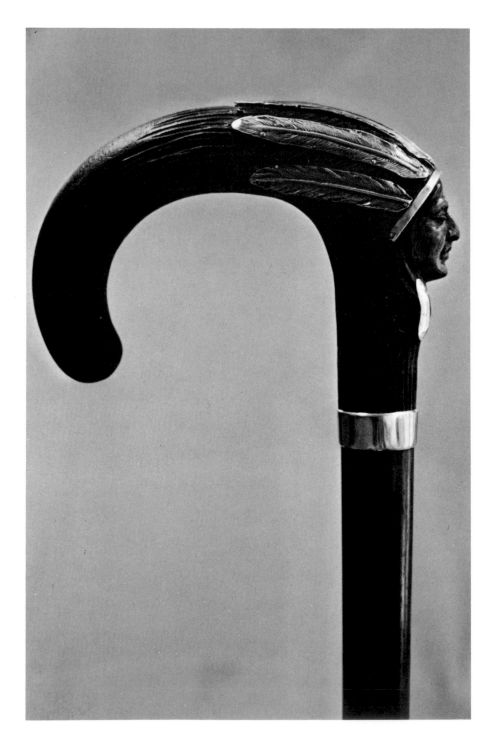

81   Female Statue of Ba-Tsho-kwe, Angola.
Statue and shaft, which is circled by a serpent,
are made from one piece. An example of rather
mediocre workmanship for this tribe, probably
from the 1930s. Not a chief's staff, but a real
walking cane. Height of figure 18 cm.

82, 83   Maori cane from New Zealand, carved
in a traditional way. A Tiki head as the end piece
and a tiki head with the typical tongue is found
in the upper third. Canes of this kind are very
rare and expensive. Auctioned on May 12, 1979
at Christie's London.

84   Baboon as handle of a walking cane of the
Ba-Rotse tribe on the Sambesi. Carved from one
piece, a piece of traditional African tribal art.
Height 11 cm.

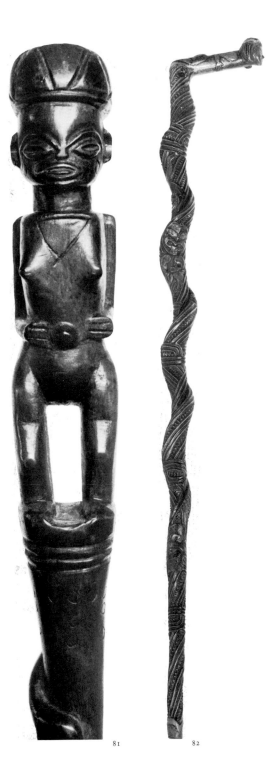

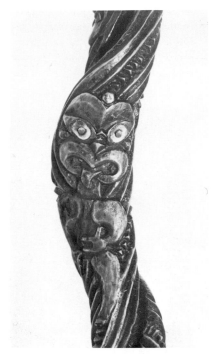

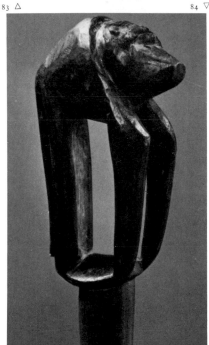

81   82   83 △   84 ▽

85-87 This cane has six faces, with six mouths, six noses, but only six eyes. Brown patinated ivory. The theme is also known to exist in silver; this, however, is definitely a copy. Renaissance or historicism period. Height 6 cm.

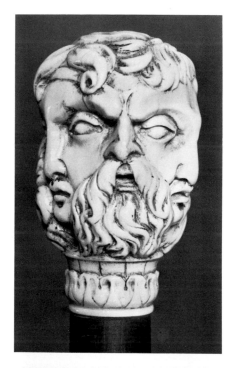

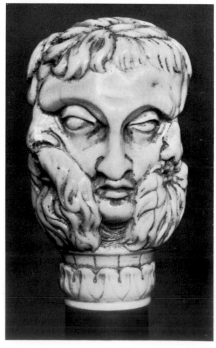

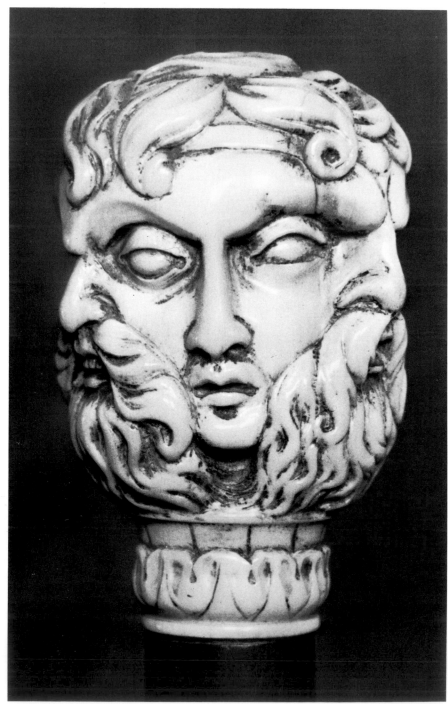

88, 89 The four male faces symbolize the black, yellow, red and white human races. Ivory, partially stained. Early 20th century.

90 T-form ivory handle with lateral maid and old man. Light red malacca shaft, a hobbyist's work. Circa early 19th century.

91 Rare pair of canes, ebony inlaid with ivory faces, carved wood frame, ivory band on shaft. Continental Europe. 18th century.

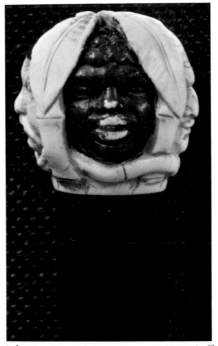

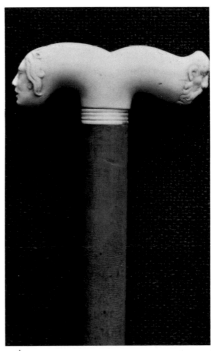

88 △   89 ▽   90 △   91 ▽

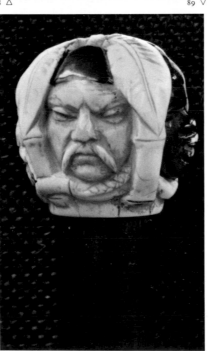

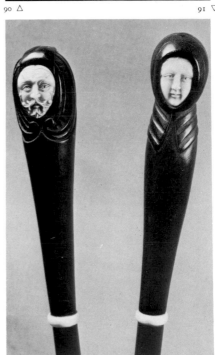

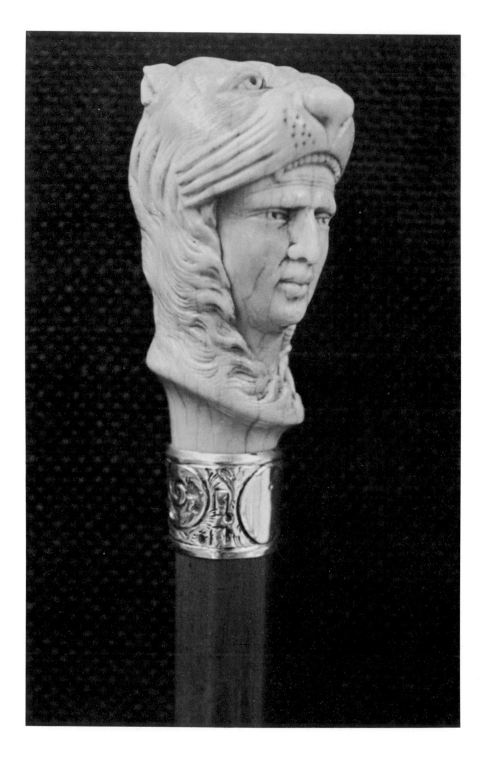

92 Hero with Lion's head and skin, probably Herakles (Hercules), frequently depicted with the skin of the mnemic lion. Antique ivory. Massive silver ring with unidentified hallmarks. England, 19th Century. Height 9 cm.

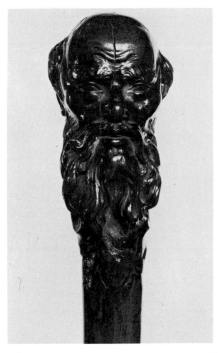

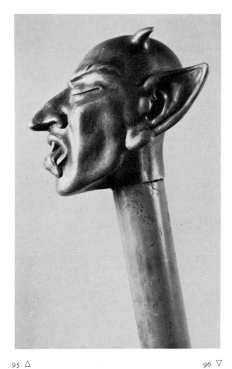

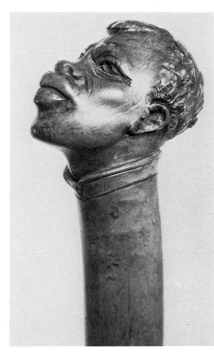

93 △   94 ▽   95 △   96 ▽   97 △   98 ▽

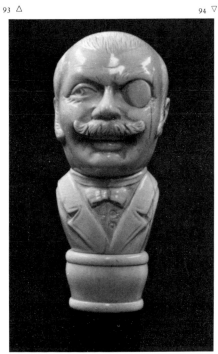

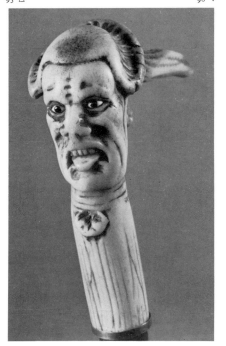

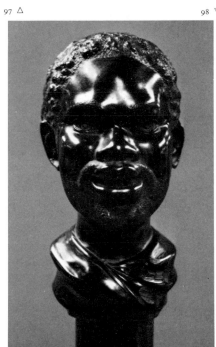

93 Male head with beard, the back of the head is carved as a lions's mask. The cane is carved from one piece. European. 17th Century. Height 12 cm.

94 Gentleman from the turn of the century with monocle. Ivory, rare, amusing work. Probably Viennese or German.

95 Satan's head in bronze. Heavy. Signed "F. Dalbiac". Around 1900.

96 Man with a grotesque face, made from a deer's antler. The antler's rose is carved as the wig. Probably late 18th Century.

97 Black's head made of hickory tree. Heavy cane made from one piece. South of the United States. Slavery period.

98 Beautiful blackamoor head, carved from dark Brazilian horn. 19th Century. Height 16 cm.

99, 100 Frederick the Great and his Greyhound are finely carved from a piece of ivory. German, 19th Century, Height 18 cm, height of figure 4.5 cm.

101 William Tell and his son, also carved in ivory. Best example of a piece from the "Historisnmus." Height 13.5 cm.

102 Bust of Napoleon in ivory, probably a period piece. Height 7 cm.

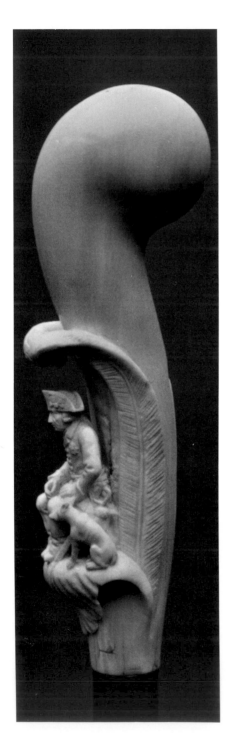

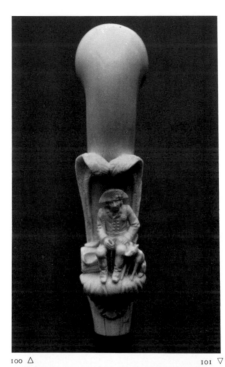

100 △   101 ▽   102 ▽

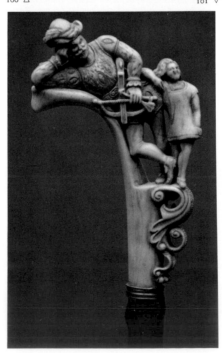

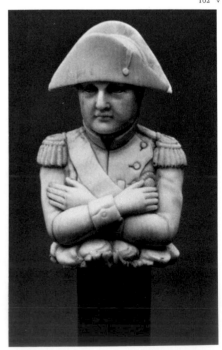

103, 104 *In England the German Kasperl is called Mister Punch and he was a common theme, sometimes together with his dog, on canes. The two illustrated ones are in sterling silver. Height 4 and 6.5 cm.*

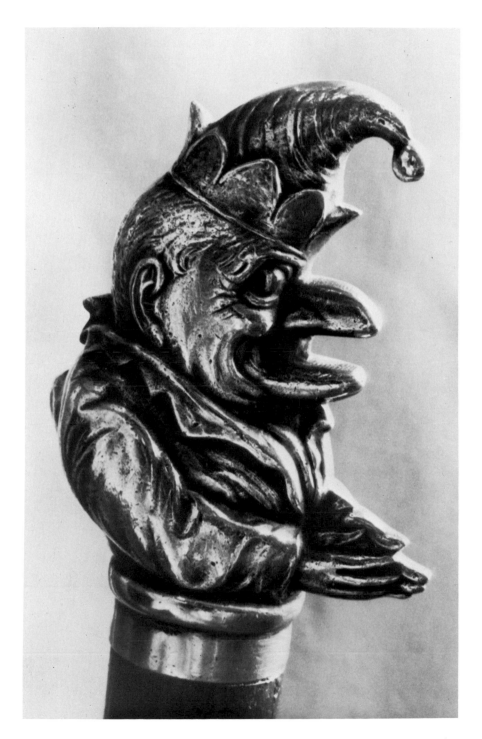

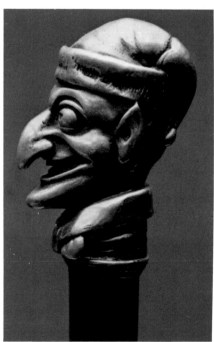

105 *Dutch merchant relieving nature. Probably Chinese ivory carving. 18th Century. Height 7.5 cm.*

106 *Emperor Wilhem with skull and serpent, winding around the cane. Colored wood, iron and brass. Signed "J. Mourtier 1914 Souvenir de siege de Verdun"*

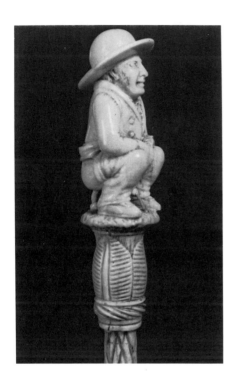

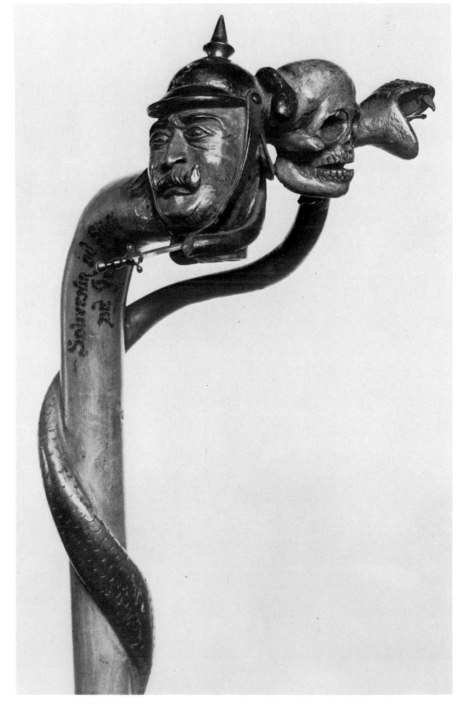

107, 108 *"Do not let yourself be fooled." Proverb cane from the Biedermeier. Ivory. Height 9 cm.*

109 *Cane with bark from one piece, carved and pierced after the design of the Ornament designed by Hieronymus von Boemmel. The wall shadow shows a greyhound. End of the 17th Century. Length 10 cm.*

110 *Turned ivory cane, the shadow image of which shows Napoleon's profile. 1814.*

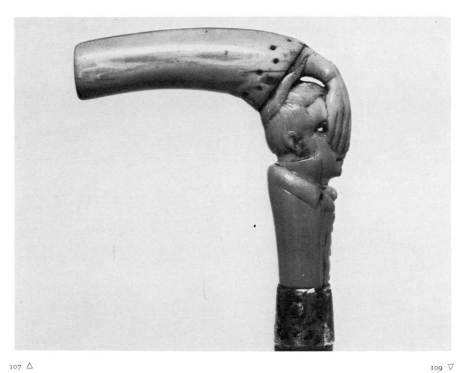

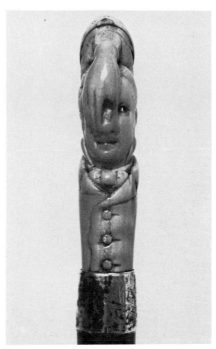

107 △   109 ▽   108 △   110 ▽

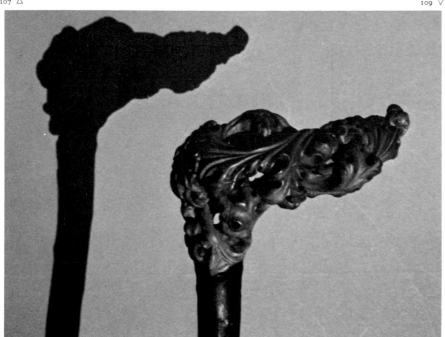

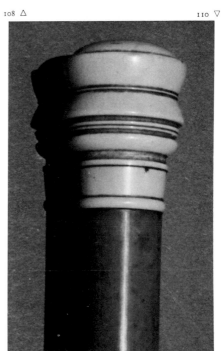

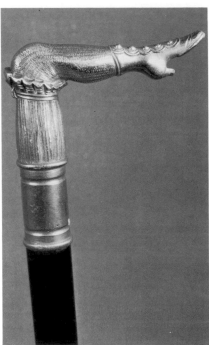

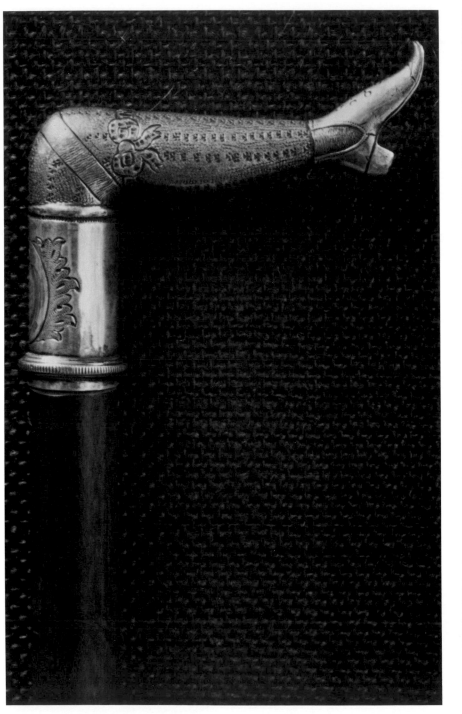

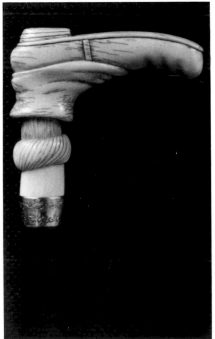

112 △   113 ▽

111, 112 *Ladies legs in stockings wearing high shoes were a favorite theme during prudish periods. Cast in metal, there canes were also used as weapons. Turn of the 20th Century.*

113 *Leg wearing stockings, shoes and gaiters, grotesque ivory cane. Probably English, turn of the 20th century. Length 9,5 cm.*

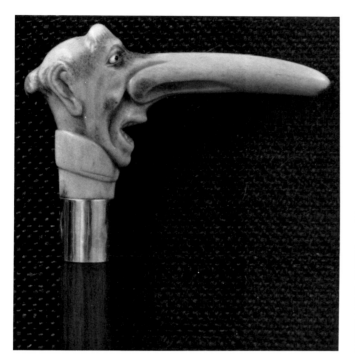

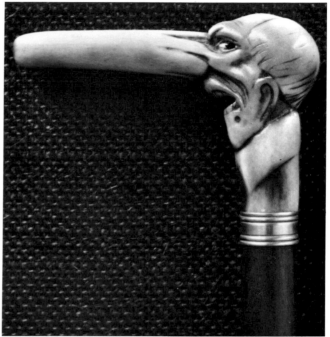

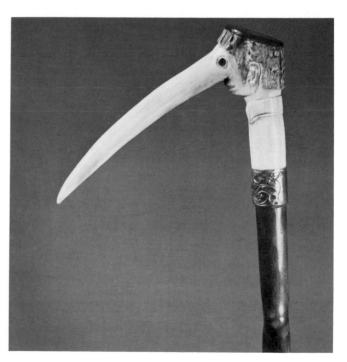

114 - 116 The "Muenchner Bilderbogen" from 1849 showed aggressive short men with long noses. The illustrations were made by Ch. Schmolze (see also illustrations 33, 46). They were the models for German canes made of deer antlers, the ends made into grotesque noses, the stronger the face the more expensive the cane. Length up to 16 cm.

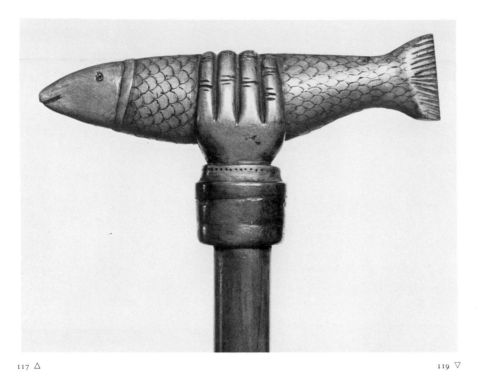

117 △

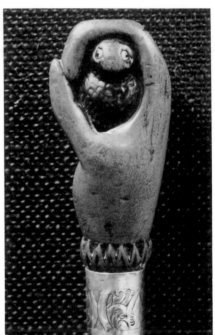

119 ▽

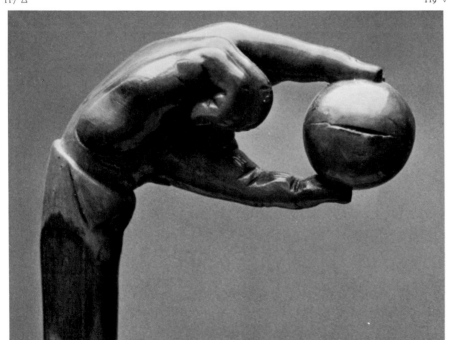

117, 118 The hand holding the fish and the hand shielding a bird are two folk art pieces from the 19th century. Length of fish 11 cm and Height of bird's hand 10 cm

119 The hand holding a ball is a reoccurring subject, done by a professional carver. Probably early 19th century.

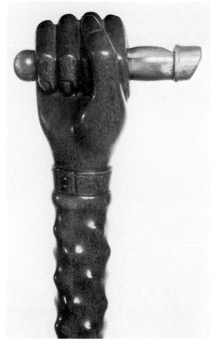

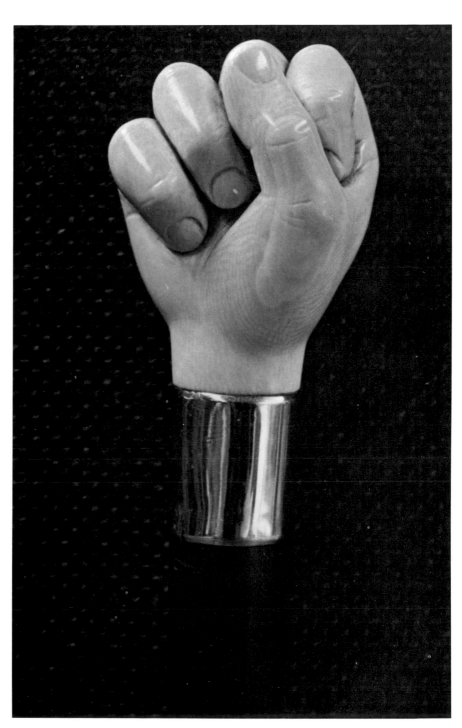

120 △   121 ▽

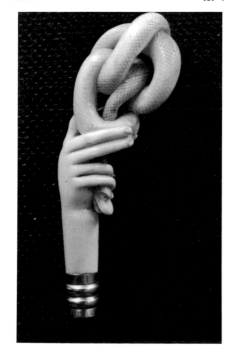

120 *A heavy rider's cane with fist and flute made from rhinoceros horn. Length 10 cm.*

121 *Hand with intertwined serpent, carved from hippopotamus tooth. Probably a lady's case. Rare subject. Middle of the 19th Century. Height of handle 10.5 cm.*

122 *Large fist made of ivory. Very well executed work from the 19th century. Height 6 cm.*

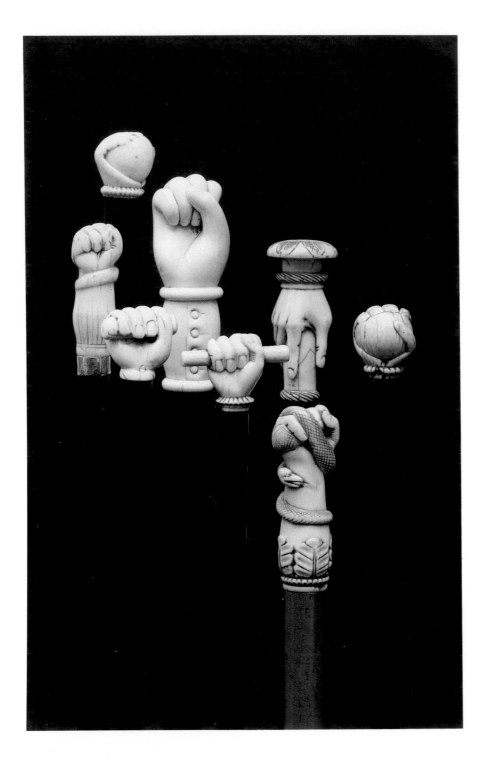

123 *The hand made into a fist is a favorite subject from the 18th Century onward. The hand either is holding a stick, a ball or a snake (height of fist with snake is 10 cm). All handles in ivory, origin usually England. The hand pointing down is probably German. The image of two intertwined hands is quite common, in colloquial language it is referred to as "hand faith."*

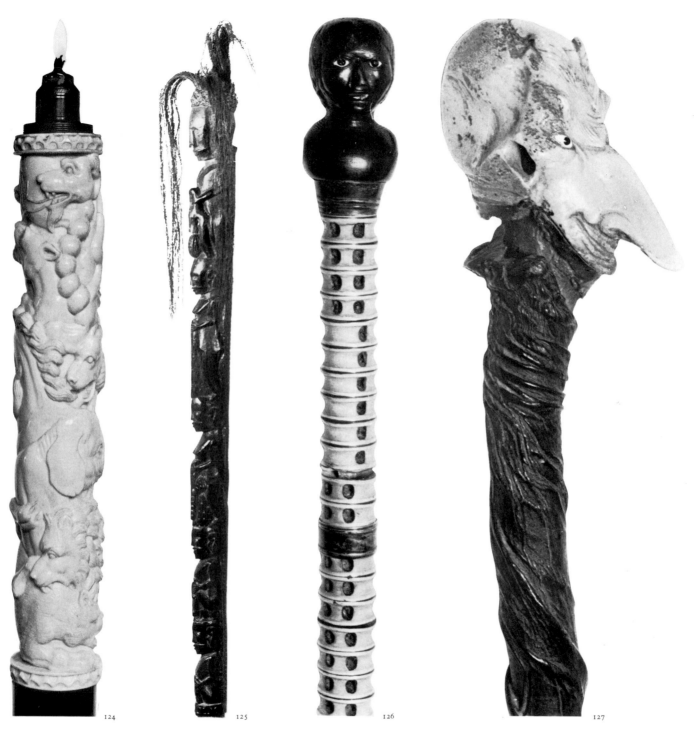

124   125   126   127

124 Battle of the animals, everybody against everybody. Probably a ceremonial cane of a secret order (black mass?). Excellent relief carving in ivory. The 21 cm long handle contains a candle, which can be concealed under a screwed ivory cap.

125 Figures one over the other ending in a rider, who has human hair wrapped around his head. Magician's cane from the Batak in Sumatra, carved from wood. Height 140 cm. The "Tondong hudjur" were sacrificed by the killing of a young boy, part of whose brain was put into an opening of the cane.

126 Magician's cane of the Voodoo priests of a Caribbean island. Made from shark's spine ending in a carved wooden female bust, having the evil eye.

127 Cane of a witch master with Satan's head, carved from the human femur and covered with human skin.

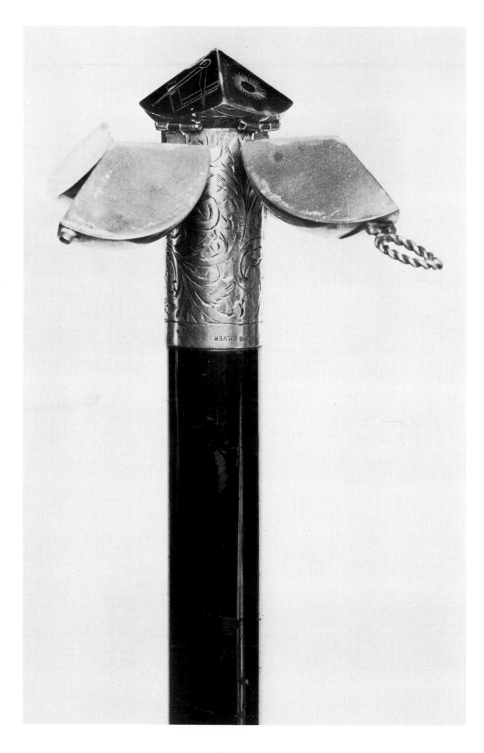

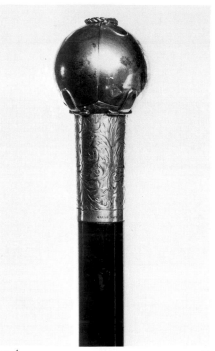

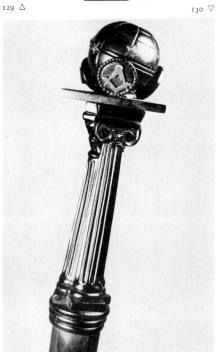

129 △   130 ▽

128, 129 *Ball or apple in silver, can be opened to reveal a pyramid with masonic emblems. Shaft is snake wood. The "Sterling" hallmark shows American origin. Diameter of ball 4 cm (illustration 128 open, illustration 129 closed)*

130 *Ball and shaft in ebony to which are applied various metal masonic emblems. The nicely turned shaft, which has a known opposite piece, is French.*

131 Skull and bones are carved from one piece of ebony. The skull has real bone teeth and is inscribed "Leperco Saint-Leger Rue d'InKermann Lille" and also bears an ankle iron, and dividers and a star within two twigs. Height of illustrated part 23 cm.

132 Skull in sterling silver, very heavy. Masonic or doctor's cane. Hallmarks London 1882. Height including neck 6.5 cm.

133 Skull with frog and serpent on pedestal. Carved from a single piece of ivory. Probably Japanese. Diameter 6 cm.

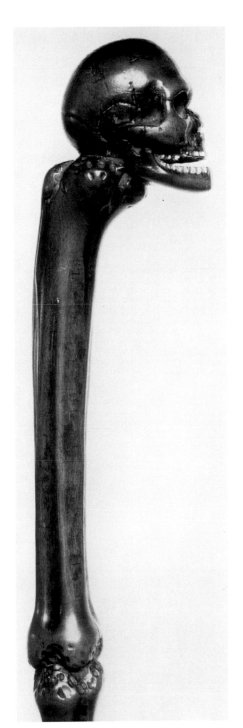

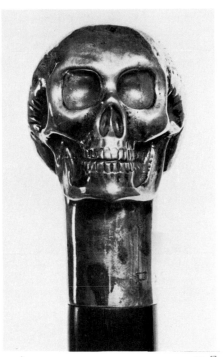

132 △

133 ▽

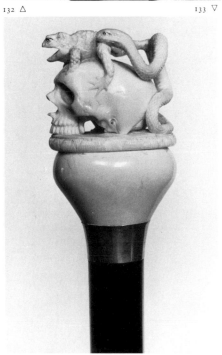

134 *The heavy, silver donkey's head is mounted on a 19 cm long piece of ivory, which contains a container for perfume. By activating a lever on the back of the head, the liquid is dispensed through an opening in the mouth. Another silver ring connects the ivory to the wooden shaft. Elegant lady's or dandy's cane. London 1904, Maker's Mark C.D. Length 8.6 cm.*

135 *Wooden Bulldog wearing a Jacobin cap, which dispenses a liquid after pushing a button. The release button is situated on the shaft and presses against a balloon. This cane may dispense stronger liquids than water (vitriol cane?)*

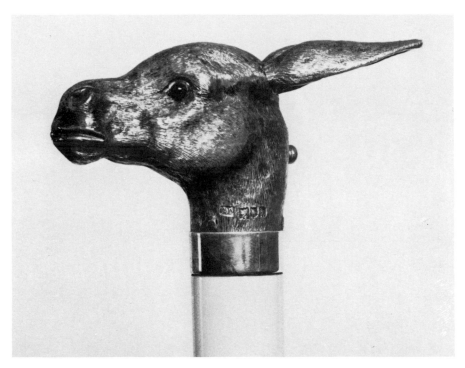

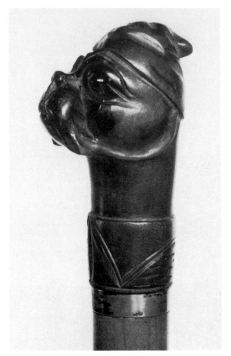

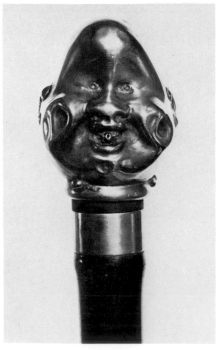

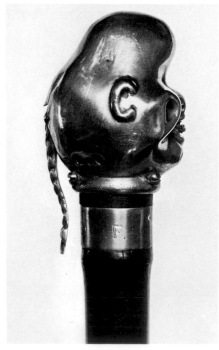

136, 137 *Chinaman's head in silver, whose pony tail serves as pump. Gag cane, to splash water. London silver marks from 1893.*

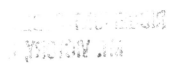

138 Upon pushing a button a skull emerges from the black ball accompanied by a clicking noise. A surprise similar to the children's toy "Jack in the Box." Diameter of the ball 4 cm.

139 Wooden donkey's head, which upon pressing of a button will wiggle his ears, and show its tongue through the opening mouth. The same donkey is also known with a simpler mechanism, mowing only its ears. Signed Louis Berthold, Bad Homburg, but probably a Viennese piece. Turn of the century. Length 8 cm.

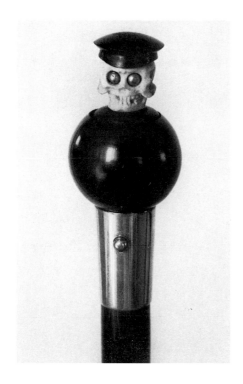

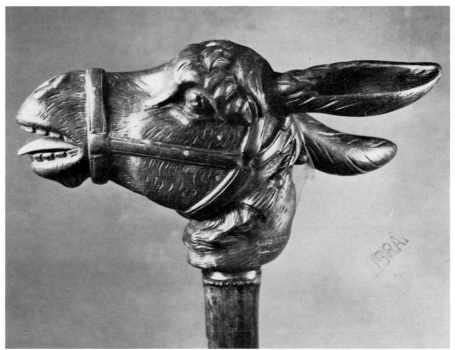

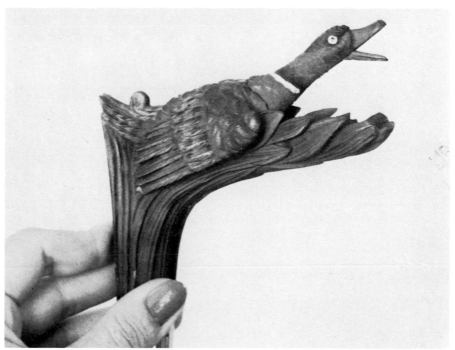

140 The duck is hidden in the rushes and appears upon pressing of a button. Very fine Viennese wood carving (see also illustration 169 of a cat).

141, 142 *Wolf with ivory release on the back. If pushed, the wolf will turn his eyes, opening his mouth, move his tongue and show well carved teeth. Tarnished ivory. Very rare model.*

143 *Bird with very long beak, which upon pushing a button opens, the tongue moves and a squeaking noise is heard. Colored ivory. Silver ring mounted by Brigg, London 1899. Made in Austria, similar to illustrations 146, 148 and 203.*

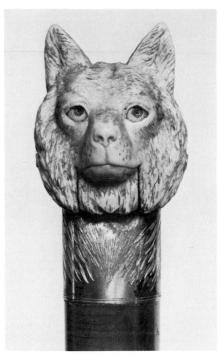

141 △   142 ▽

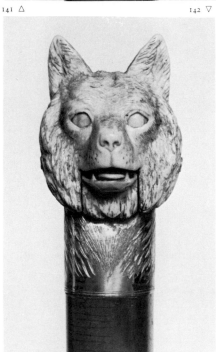

143 ▽

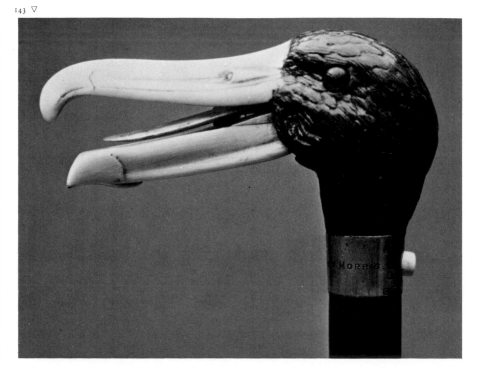

144, 145 Wooden dog, with a button on the back of the head. He can turn his eyes and show his red tongue.

146, 147 Donkey made of colored ivory, can move his ears and open his mouth, showing a pink colored tongue. Brigg, London 1896.

148, 149 Ivory cockatoo, with multi-colored feathers, can open the polished beak and make a sound. Rare flirt cane. Brigg, London 1898.

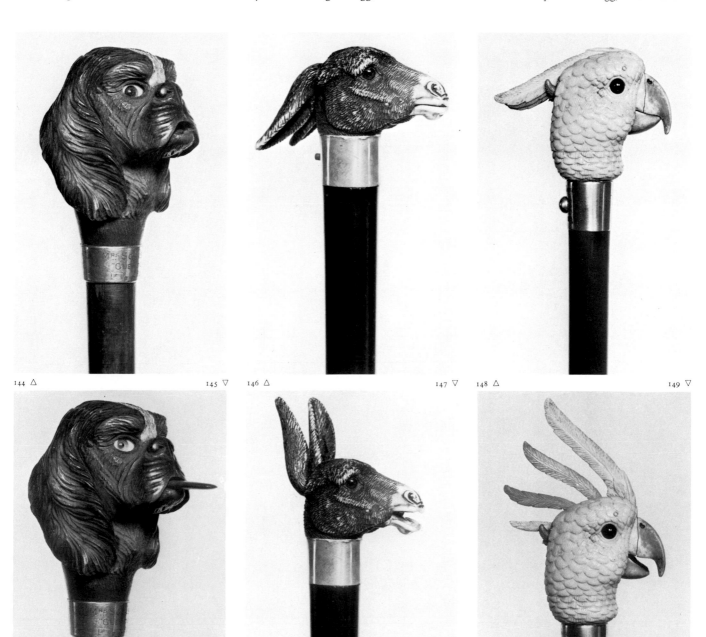

144 △   145 ▽   146 △   147 ▽   148 △   149 ▽

150, 151 The monkey is a popular automaton with numerous variations; the one illustrated is wearing a cap, turns his multi-colored eyes, opens his mouth and sticks his tongue out. Head and band in ivory.

152, 153 Monk's head in ivory, turning his eyes, opening his mouth and sticking his tongue out. Hallmark London 1884, Maker's Mark JD. Engraved inscription (Maker/) "H.M. Emanuel & Son/Portsea." Height of head 5.5 cm.

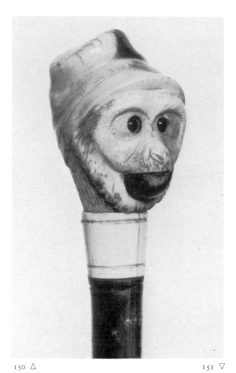

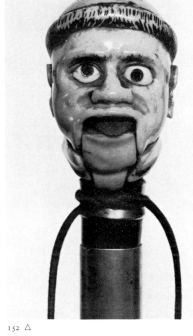

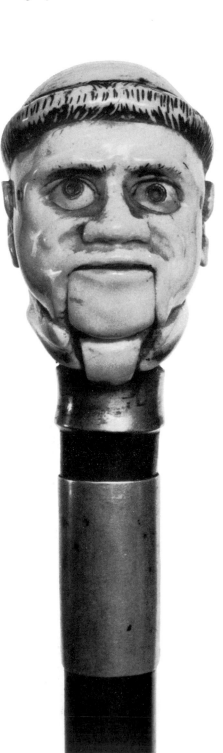

150 △   151 ▽   152 △   153 ▷

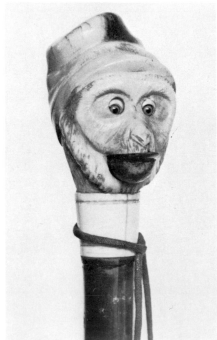

154, 155 *Blackamoor head in wood, rolls ivory eyes at the push of a button, opens the mouth and sticks his red tongue out.*

156, 157 *Fat, friendly monk in ivory who, upon pushing a button, turns his eyes toward the sky and opens his mouth in a smile.*

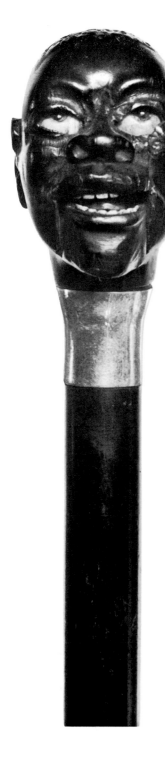

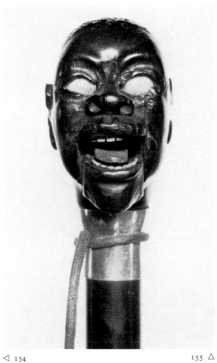

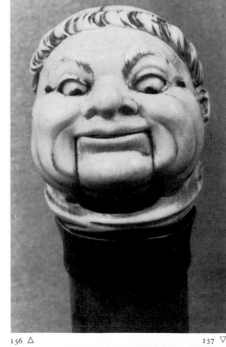

◁ 154   155 △   156 △   157 ▽

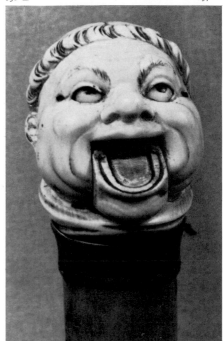

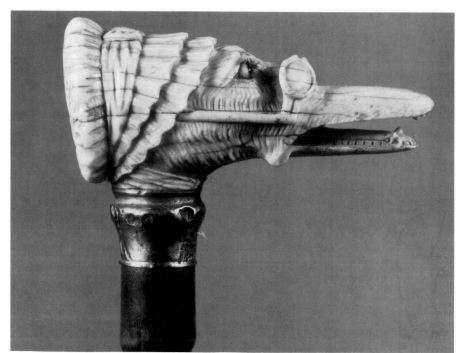

158 Goose with cap and glasses, finely carved in ivory. Probably after the old children's tale "Mother Goose," which was illustrated in 1881 by Kate Greenaway. The "Scenes de la vie privee et publique des animaux" might have also been a model. Second half of the 19th century.

158 △   159 ▽   160 ▽

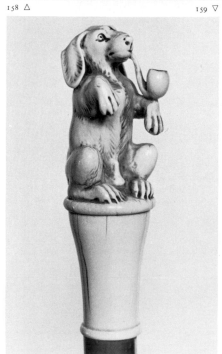

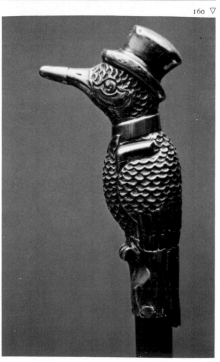

159 Dog standing on its hind legs (dachshund or basset), with an ivory pipe. Continental Europe, turn of the 20th century. Height of figure only 6.5 cm.

160 Woodpecker with top hat, collar, tie and cane (bird's wedding), low carat silver. Height 11 cm.

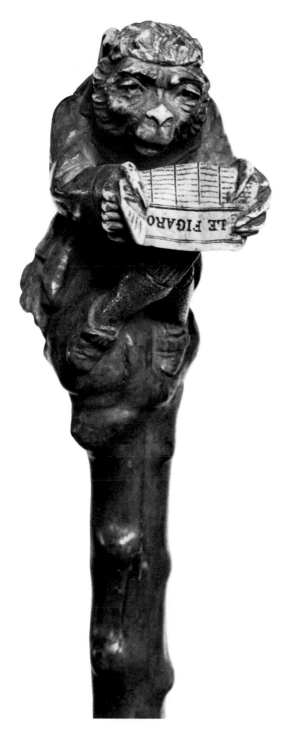

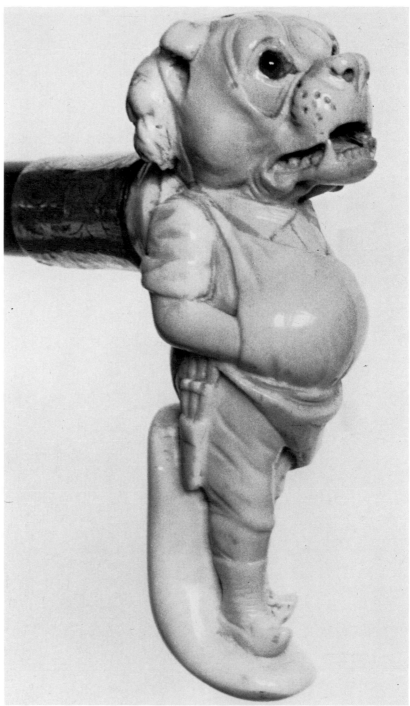

161 "The Monkey Reading Le Figaro" after a lithograph by Honore Daumier, finely carved in nut wood and ivory. Head, hands, paper and tail are made of ivory. Riding cane from one piece of wood. French, 2nd half of the 19th century. Height of figure 7 cm.

162 Bulldog as cook or butcher, with apron and hat. Well executed ivory carving. Handle in the style of Grandville. Probably French, middle of 19th century, Length 12 cm.

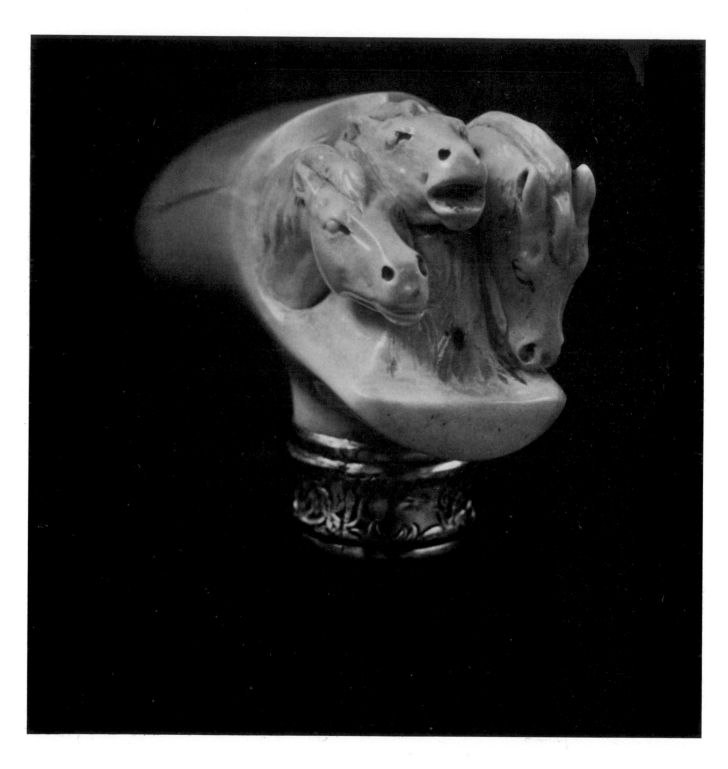

163   *Three horses racing head next to head, emerging from the tip of an elephant's tusk. Probably turn of the 20th century. Length 15 cm.*

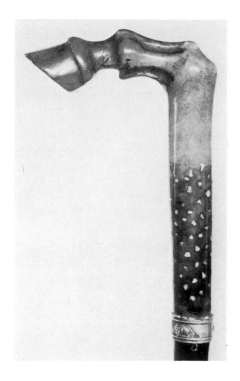

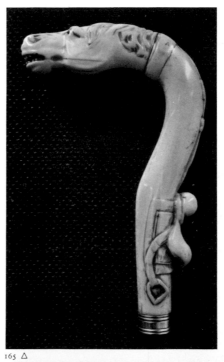

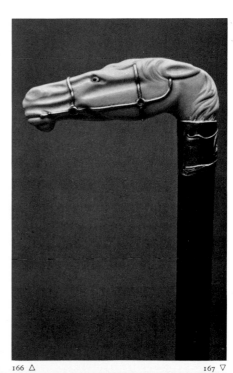

165 △   166 △   167 ▽

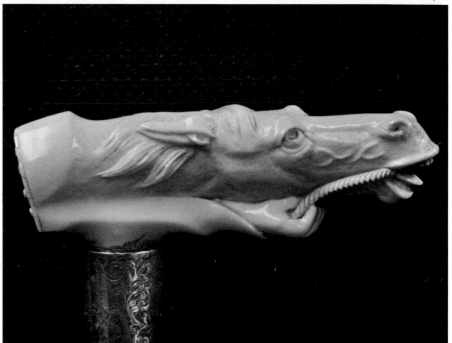

164 Horseshoe and leg, a favored cane motif, are in tortoise with mother of pearl inlay. Probably German. Height 13 cm.

165 Very expressive head of a horse, with saddle, stirrups and cap at the base. In two parts, made from hippopotamus tooth. Right handed. Probably English. 19th Century. Height 15 cm.

166 Horse's head with bridle, made from silver thread.

167 Horse's head with hand grabbing the snaffle. The handle ending in a horse shoe. Probably English. Length 14 cm.

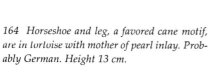

168 Wooden cat with automated ears and mouth (glove holder). Typical Viennese work from about 1900. The shaft holds a sword. Height of knob 7 cm.

169 Very finely carved wooden cat, which, upon pushing a button, can turn its head and lift its tail, from Vienna. Height 13.5 cm.

170 Cat sitting on a branch lurking above two mice. Made of ivory. Probably English, around 1900. Height 12 cm.

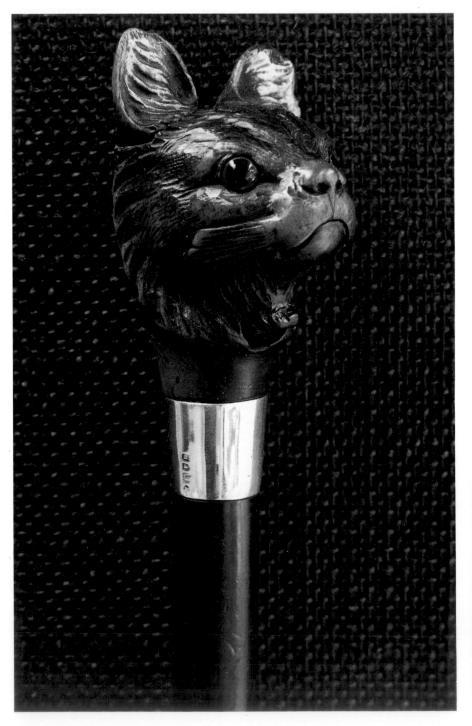

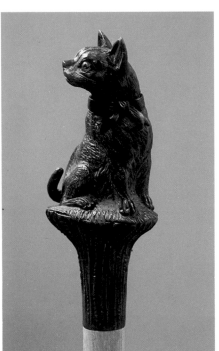

169 △   170 ▽

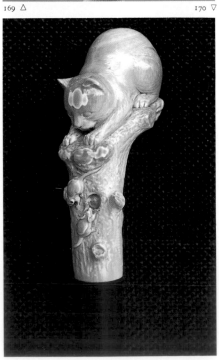

171 Two rats, playing with an egg. Ivory, Japanese work. Original cane handle, not a converted Netsuke.

172 Heads of mice are carved all over the handle, which has a cat's heads at each end. The eye's of the mice are set with red rhinestones. Probably Victorian. Length 12.5 cm.

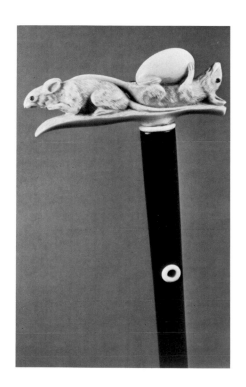

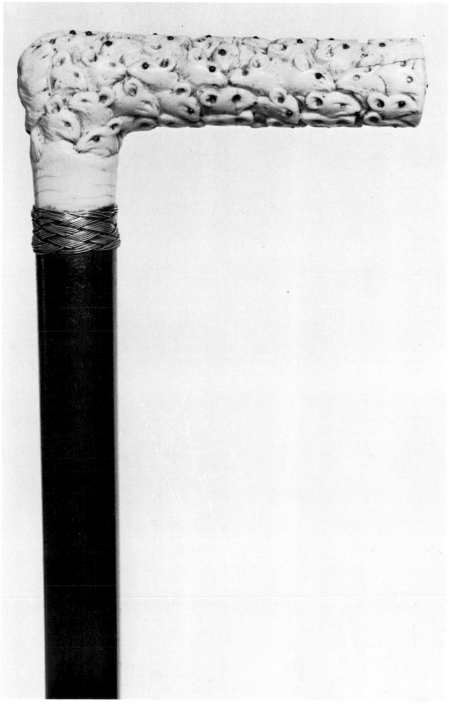

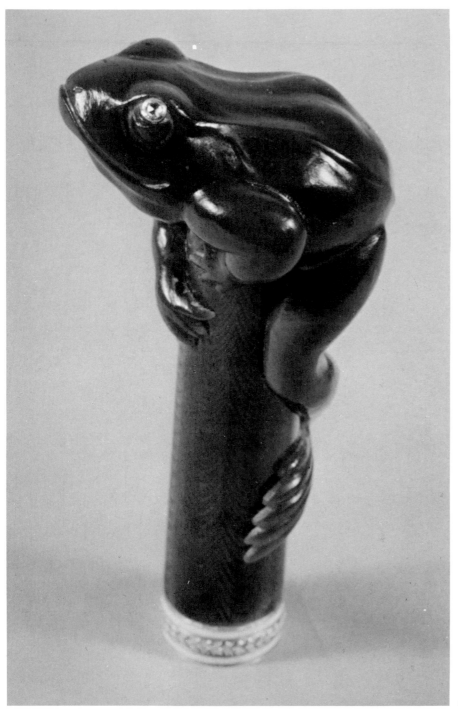

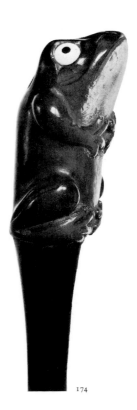

173 Nephrite frog, mounted green enameled gold column by Henrik Wigstroem, from the atelier of Carl Fabergé, Petersburg. Unmounted. Turn of the 20th century. Height 11.5 cm.

174 Painted wooden frog with large eyes and feet placed on its stomach. Height 9 cm.

173   174

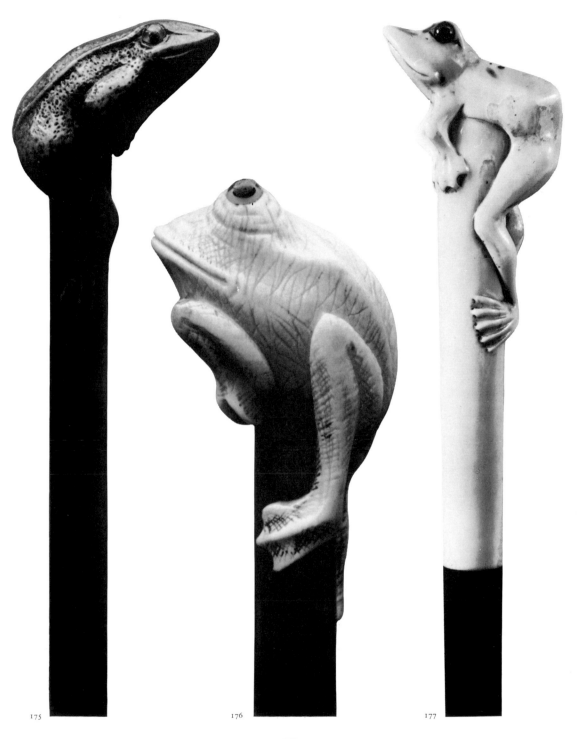

175   176   177

175-177 *These three frogs climbed up the walking sticks, the two on the right are from Japan. 175 wooden frog, Height 5 cm. 176 Bull frog, ivory. Height 7 cm. 177 Tree frog, ivory, Height 6 cm.*

178 Wooden bear chained to a tree. Handle and shaft carved from one piece. Probably Swiss (The bear from Bern), last third of the 19th Century.

179 Minutely carved donkey's head in hardwood. Most likely Viennese, despite the Birmingham Mark from 1896 on the silver band. Length 10.5 cm.

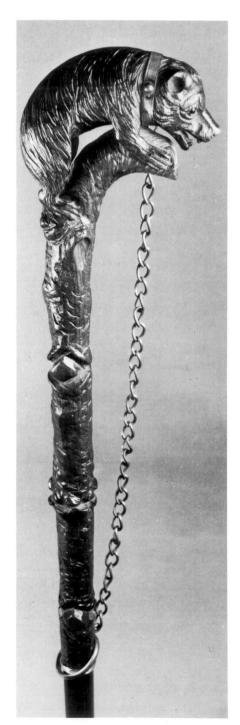

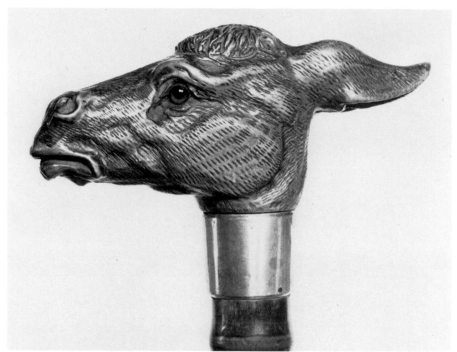

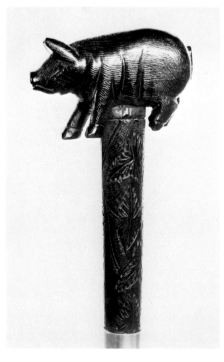

180 Piglet carved from black thorn, mounted on black thorn shaft. The upper portion of the shaft carved with black thorn leaves and berries, clover and a harp in relief. Ireland, 19th Century, Length of handle 8 cm.

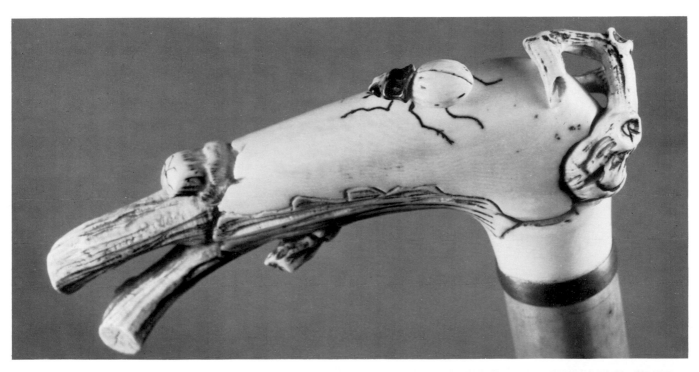

181 Stylized root with beetle, stained in red and black. Ivory. France, 19th Century, after a Chinese model.

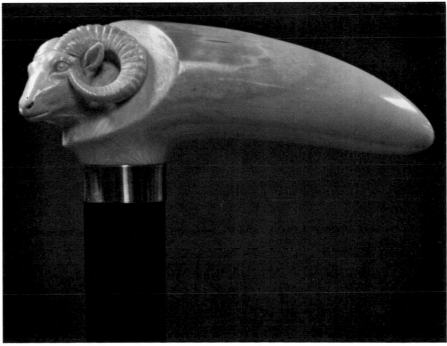

182 Ram's head, carved out of the tip of an elephant's tusk. Heavy handle with nice patina. Length 13 cm.

183   Rabbit, sitting in beets, carved from the tip of an elephant's tusk. Very fine English work, very decorative, 19th Century, Length 14.5 cm.

184   A rabbit is coming out of a shepherd's leg crook. Ivory, England, 19th Century.

185   Jumping rabbit in ivory. Unusual image. The handle fits well into the hand. Probably English, around 1900. Length 13.5 cm.

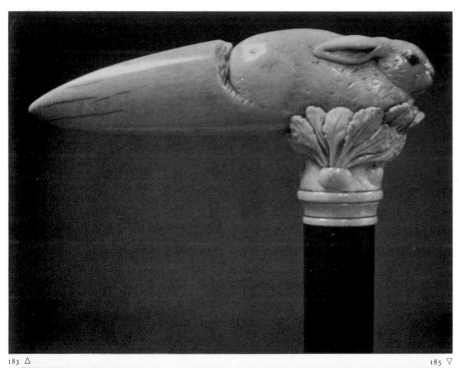

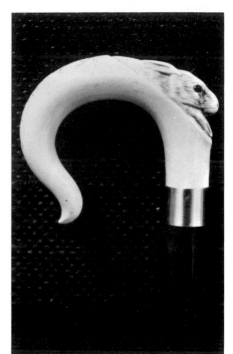

183 △   185 ▽

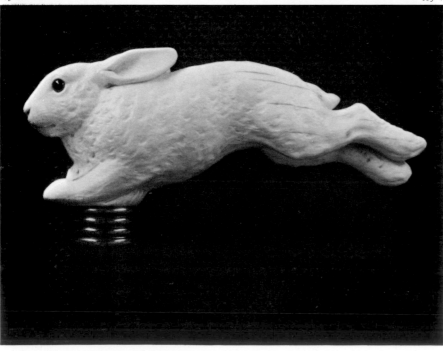

186 Hare's head with brown glass eyes. White ivory. The collar suggests, that the image might be the "White Rabbit" from "Alice in Wonderland." The craftsmen made several models with identical subject. England(?) Turn of the 20th Century(?). Length 13 cm.

187 Finely carved wooden rabbit in the Viennese style. The gold band is 9 k gold with English hallmarks and the inscription "EMG from JG." Length 8 cm.

188 Rabbit with ears put up, in ivory. Probably England, circa 1900. Height 8.5 cm.

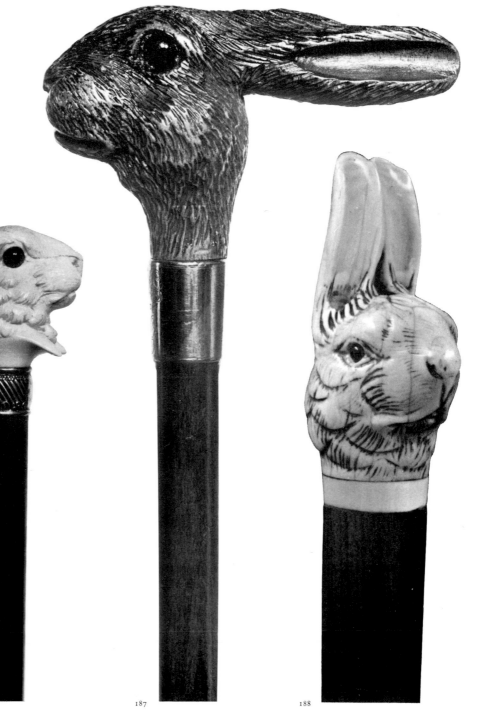

186   187   188

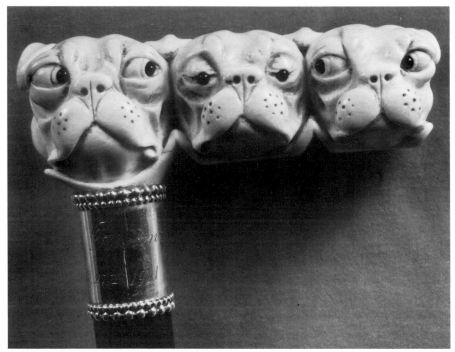

189 Three pugs in ivory. The two outer ones care-
fully observing the resting one in the middle.
Amusing handle. Probably early 20th century.
Length 10 cm.

189 △   190 ▽   191 ▽

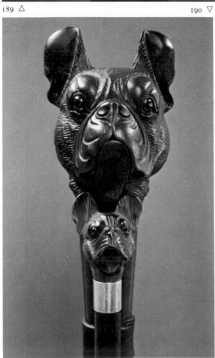
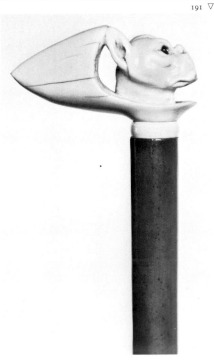

190 Bulldog head glove holder carved in wood.
The one in front has regular size, the one in the
back is 26 cm high. Probably a display cane for a
store.

191 Bull dog, carved from pottwhale tooth. Well
patinated. Length 8.5 cm.

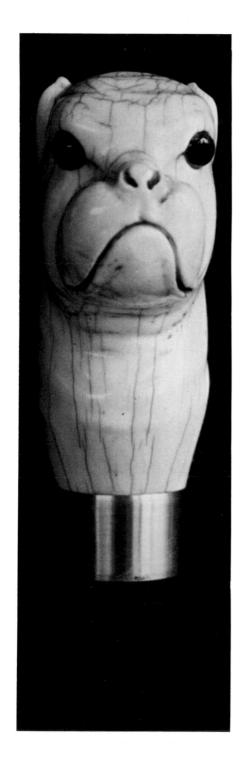

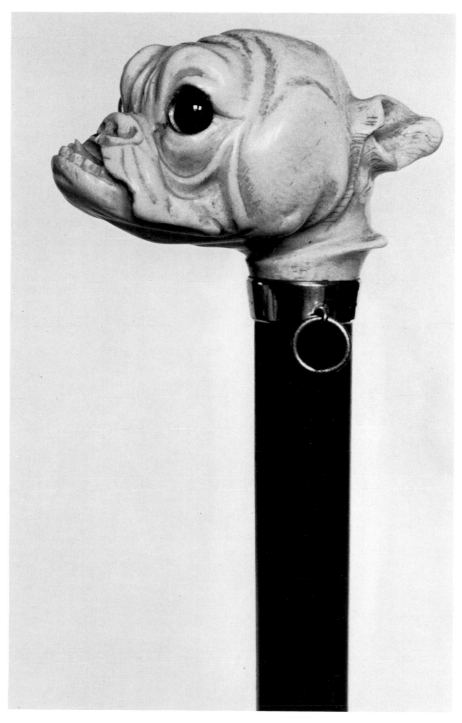

192 Stylized mastiff in pale cracked ivory, un-
usually massive. Probably English. 2nd Half
19th Century. Height 10.5 cm.

193 Naturalistic Boxer with extended lower jaw, ivory, gold
band with ring as collar. Excellent work, probably by an English carver whose carving style is identifiable. Other examples
of his work exist. Length 9 cm.

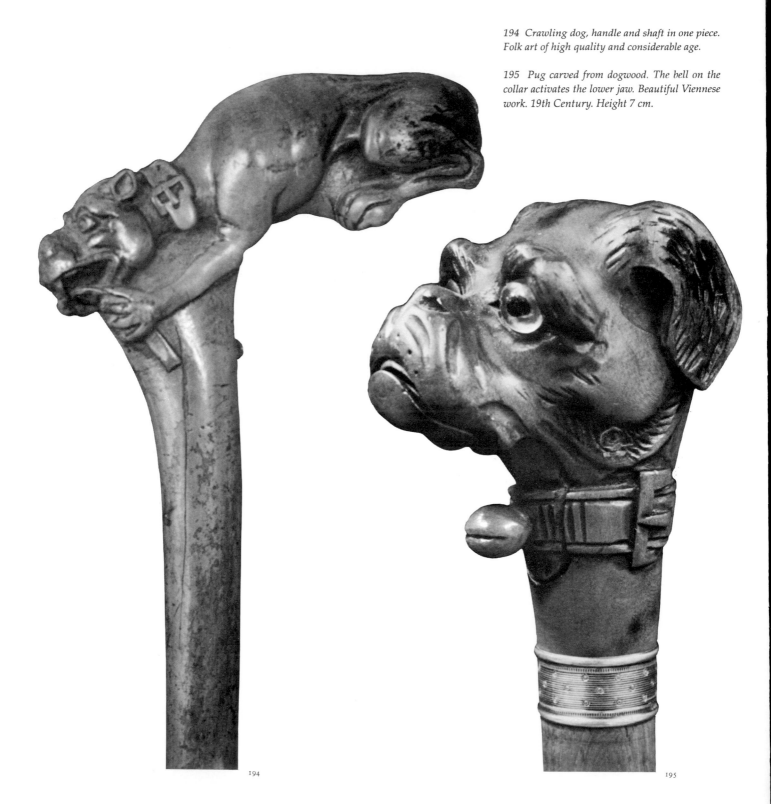

194 Crawling dog, handle and shaft in one piece. Folk art of high quality and considerable age.

195 Pug carved from dogwood. The bell on the collar activates the lower jaw. Beautiful Viennese work. 19th Century. Height 7 cm.

194

195

196 A finely carved ivory Spaniel is laying on the rose of a deer antler. The ivory band is carved with resting deer. Excellent Viennese work. 19th Century, Height 6.5 cm.

197 Simple hunting cane with carved dog's head in hardwood on chestnut wood shaft. German. Height 10.5 cm.

198 Excellent carving of a poodle in ivory, very lively. Ivory mounted on leather disc shaft. France.

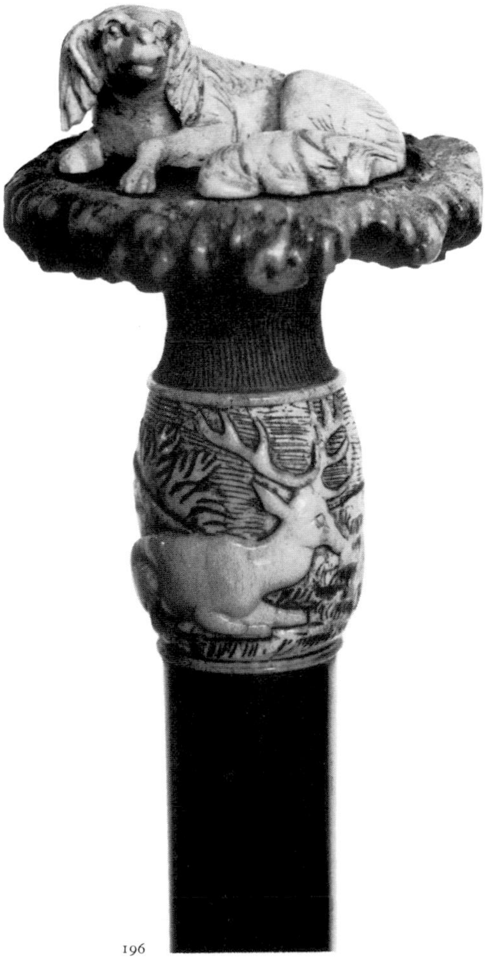

196

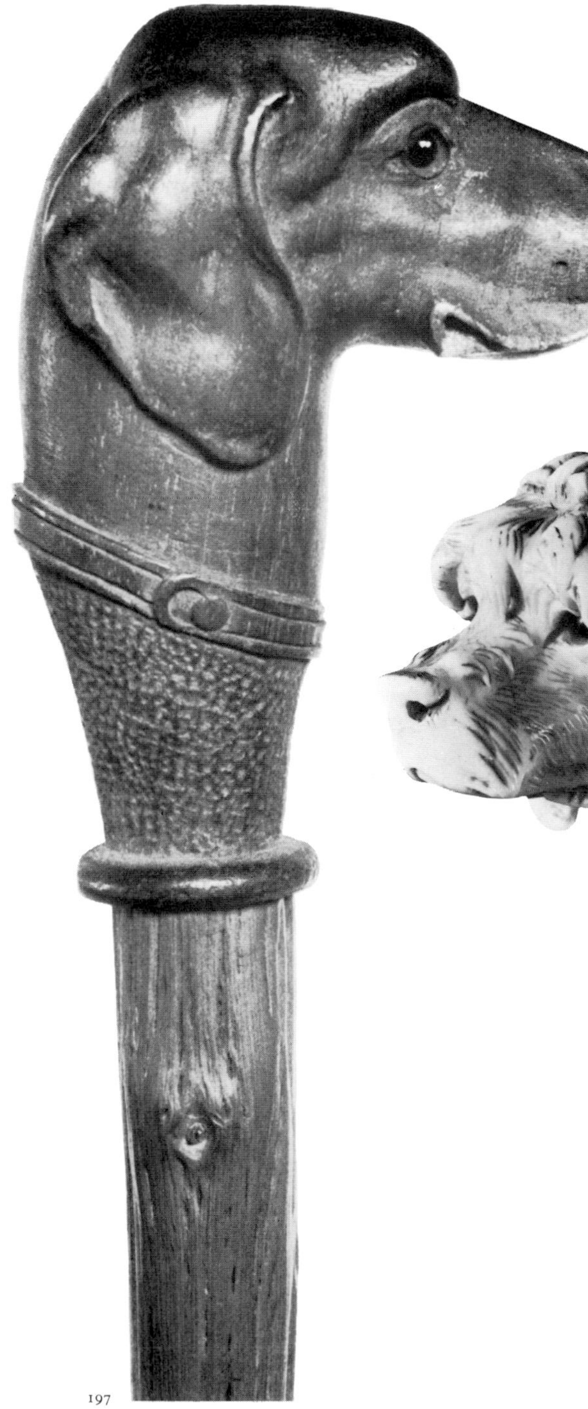

197

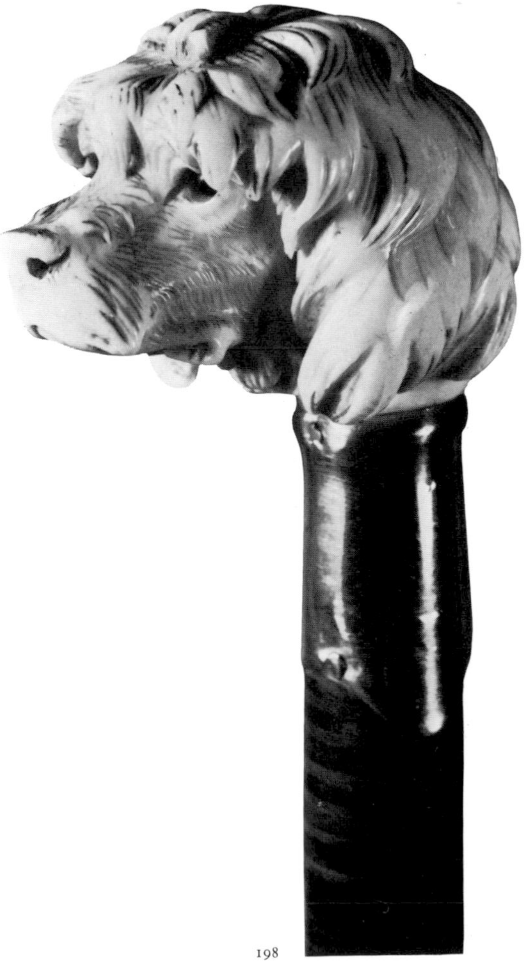

198

199 *Massive dog's head with large teeth, holding a giant bone, which forms the handle. Ivory carving. Unusual continental European piece. 2nd half 19th Century. Length 13 cm.*

200 *Large mastiff dog's head in ivory with muzzle in silver thread. Original and impressive piece. Band and collar in silver. England (?). Length 7 cm.*

201 *Opera style handle with boxer head from hippopotamus tooth. Beautiful tan patina and nerve seam (see page 224), floral silver band. Probably English.*

202 *Wooden boxer head, carved as crook handle. Ears, eye brows, nose and teeth inlaid in ivory. A frequent model in different qualities of execution. Probably German, around 1900.*

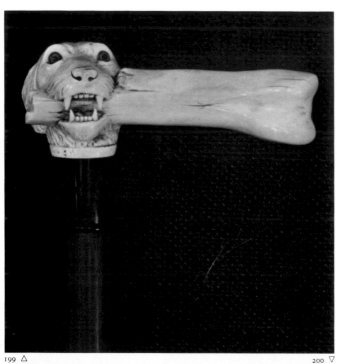

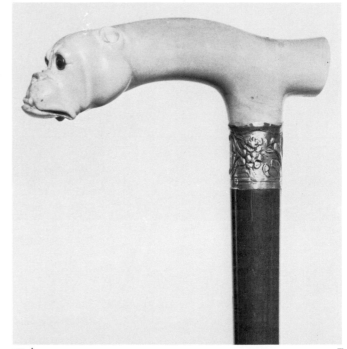

199 △   200 ▽   201 △   202 ▽

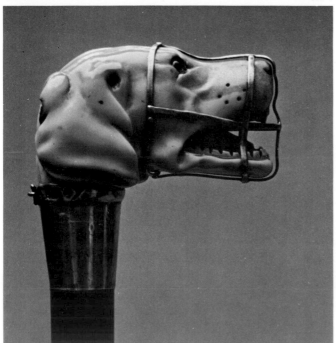

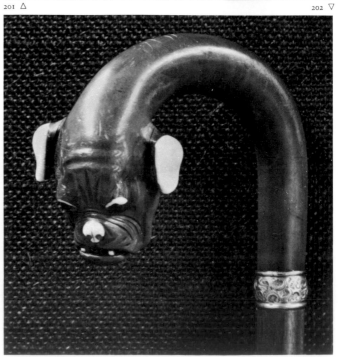

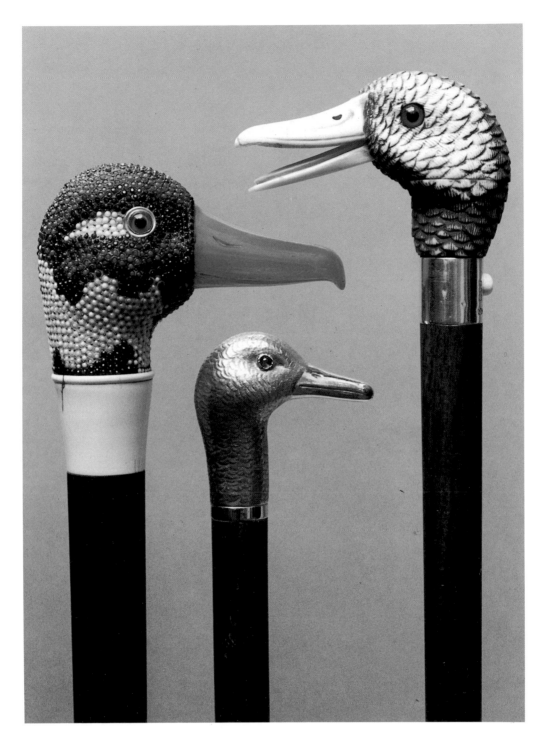

203 From left: Beak and eyes are made of horn, with applied glass beads as feathers. The shine is even further increased by applied brass nails. Length 9.5 cm. Two ounces of 18 k gold and sapphire eyes were used for this duck's head. Made in 1902 by Charles Cook for Brigg in London. — This colored ivory duck was made for the same retailer. Upon pushing a button the beak opens and the tongue moves to a quacking sound.

204 *Parrot cleaning his feathers, while sitting on the cane with his tail feathers folding around it. Ivory with horn beak. Beautiful work from the 1920s. 20th Century. Height 11 cm.*

205 *Squatting ivory parrot. A lovely handle which fits well into the hand: a walking stick.*

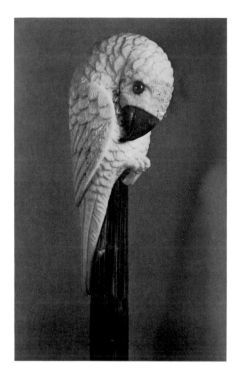

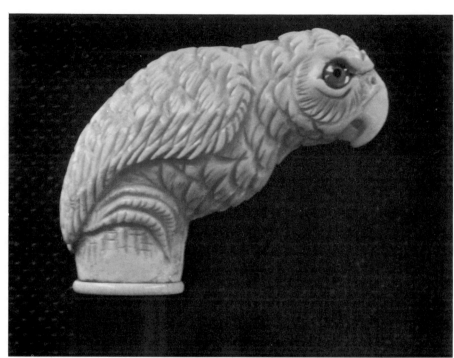

206 *Stylized toucan roughly carved from a wart-hog tooth. Probably English, 19th century. Length of tooth on the longer side 33 cm.*

207 *Large deer antler fork, with silver eagle's head at base. Iron shaft. Custom-made piece for hunter. Probably German, Length 26 cm.*

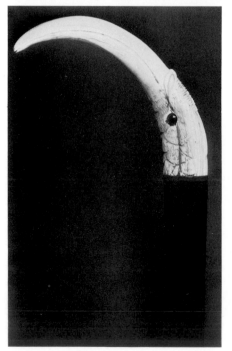

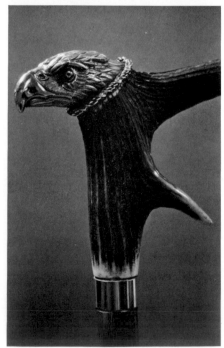

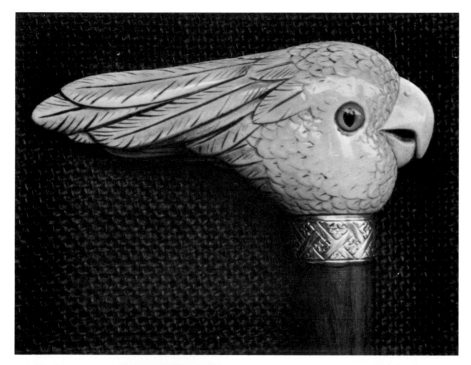

208 *Bird's head from the parrot family, carved ivory with color stains. Exclusive and diligently made piece by Brigg, London, circa 1890. Length 12 cm.*

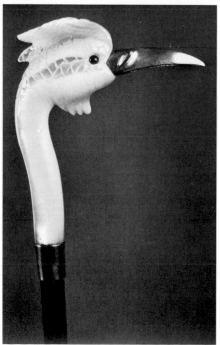

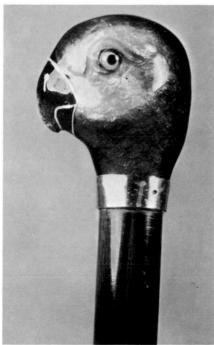

209 *Heron, mother of pearl carving with silver beak. Very fine lady's cane. Probably French, circa 1890.*

210 *Parrot's head in multi-color enamel. Continental European. Height 4.5 cm.*

211 *Owl, sitting on a rock, with large mother of pearl eyes, carved in ebony. Japanese. 2nd Half 19th Century. Signed "Moto Tsuku." Height 7.5 cm.*

212 *Ivory elephant laying on its stomach and laughing. Naive and amusing carving. Probably Indian, end of the 19th century. Length 11 cm.*

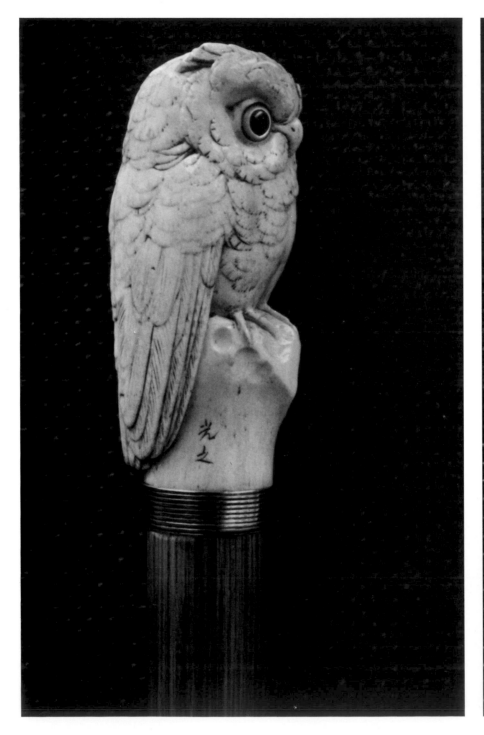

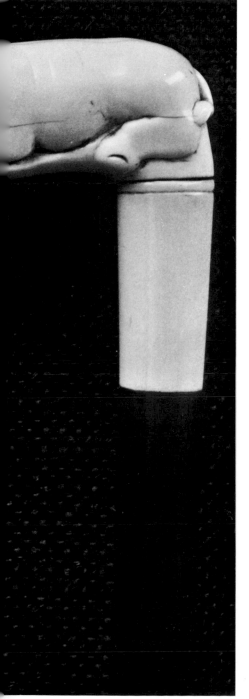

213 *Ivory elephant balancing on a globe, with English silver marks. Illustration in actual size.*

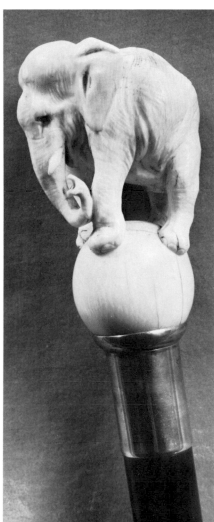

214 *Elephant tower. Very fine Japanese piece in tinted ivory. 2nd half 19th Century. Height 14 cm.*

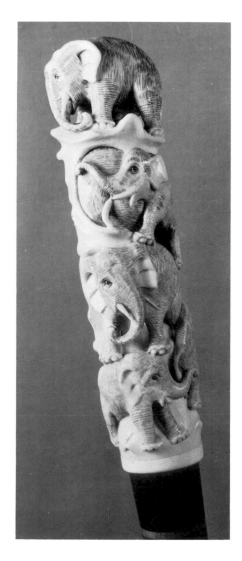

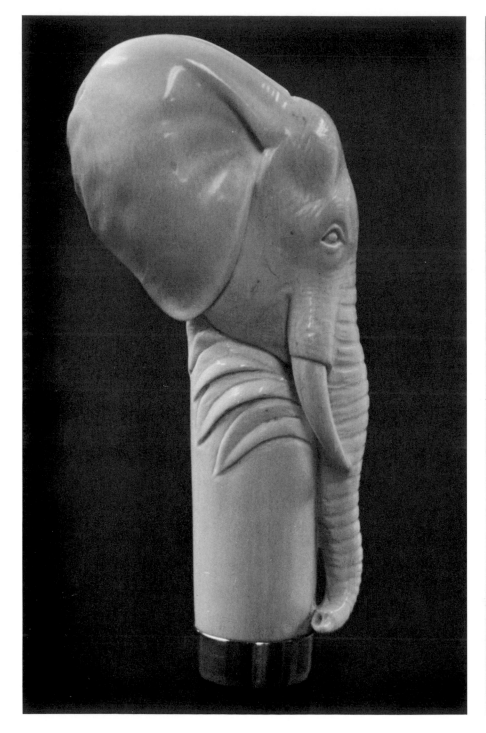

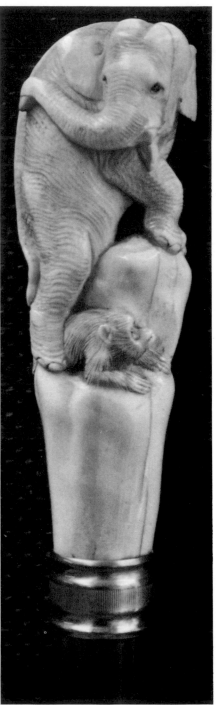

215 *Large head of an African elephant with ears laying alongside head and palm leaf decoration. Ivory. European carving. Late 19th Century. Height 10 cm.*

216 *Elephant, standing on a rock, is harassed by two monkeys. Japanese work of exceptional beauty and naturalistic quality. End of 19th century. Height 10 cm.*

217 *Elephant's head, finely carved in siam horn, the tusks in ivory. Unusual and elegant cane, the trunk forming the crook handle.*

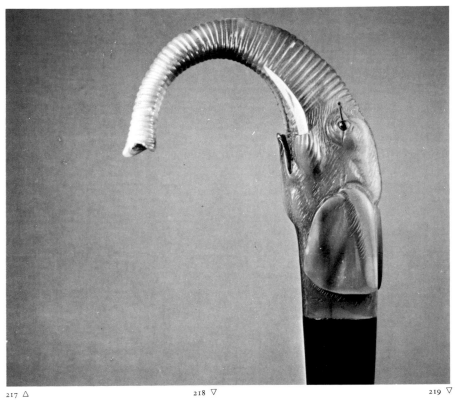

217 △

218, 219 *Ivory elephant carved into a ball form, partially tinted. Amusing Japanese work, most likely by a netsuke carver, but made as a cane handle. This model appears several times in different sizes. Diameter 5 cm.*

218 ▽

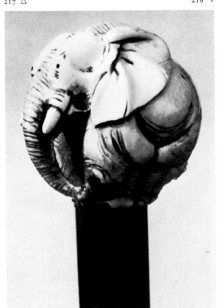

219 ▽

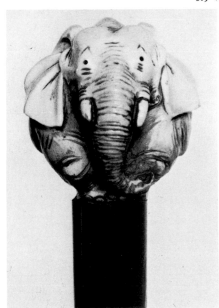

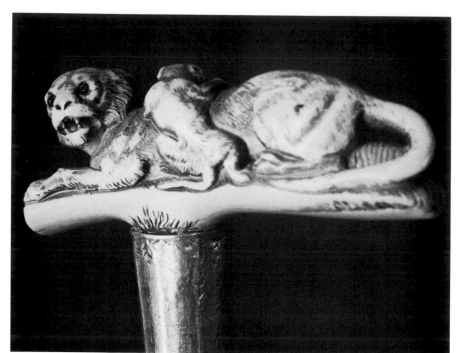

220 Female lion with cub. Ivory carved in a way that the bottom plate allows for a good handle. 18th Century (?)

220 △

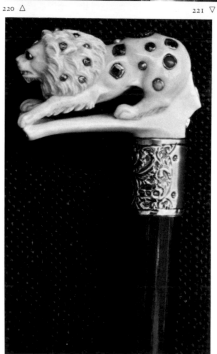

221 ▽

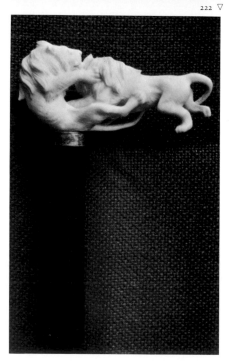

222 ▽

221 Parading ivory lion, applied with 34 k gold set gem stones: sapphires, rubies, emeralds, diamonds, topaz, turquoise, opal and pearls. Made for an Indian Maharadscha after models from the Middle Ages. With original fitted box. Birmingham, 1894. Length 8 cm.

222 Two fighting ivory lions. Probably far eastern, very distinguished piece for the European market.

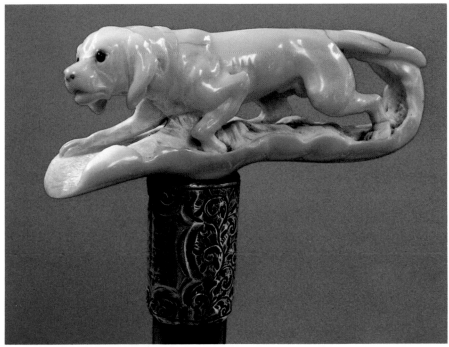

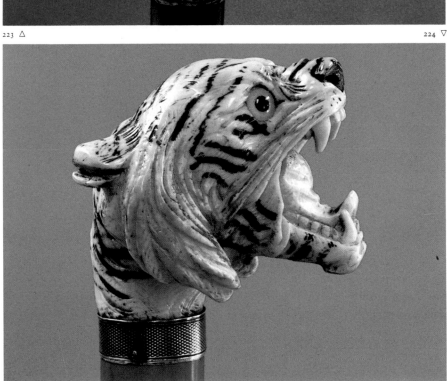

223 △   224 ▽

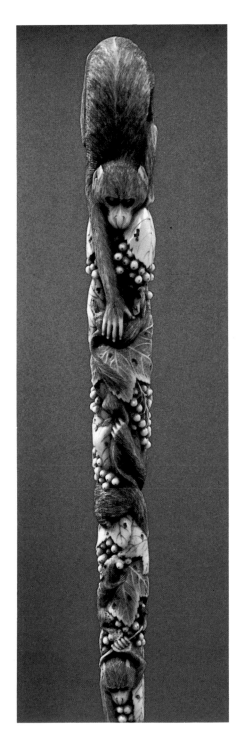

223 Well patinated ivory hunting dog. The base plate forms a well fitting handle for the left hand. The English inscription from 1897 corresponds with the Birmingham silver mark. The very lively dog seems to be German made. Length 10 cm.

224 Unusual Tiger's head with open mouth, naturalistically stained ivory. Japan(?) Height 6 cm.

225 Monkeys stealing fruit is a favored subject in Japan. The ivory is stained and very finely carved. An example of excellent Japanese work, which makes Japanese crafts so desirable. Height 32 cm.

226 *The female lion has grabbed the serpent which is wound around a tree. Finely executed ivory carving by an artist or a work shop which has executed this theme in many ways. 19th Century. Height 9 cm.*

227 *The serpent is climbing toward the bear. Simple yet charming ivory carving. Height 8 cm.*

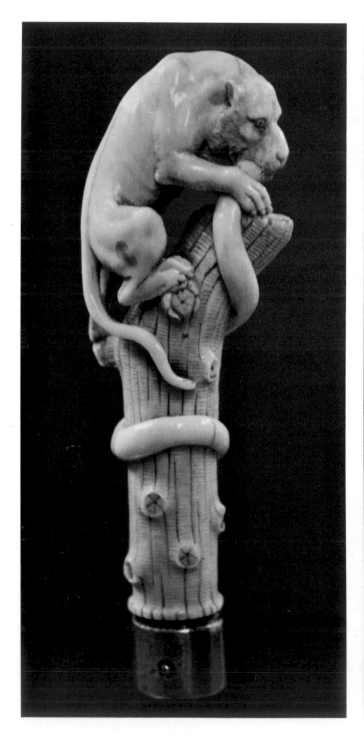

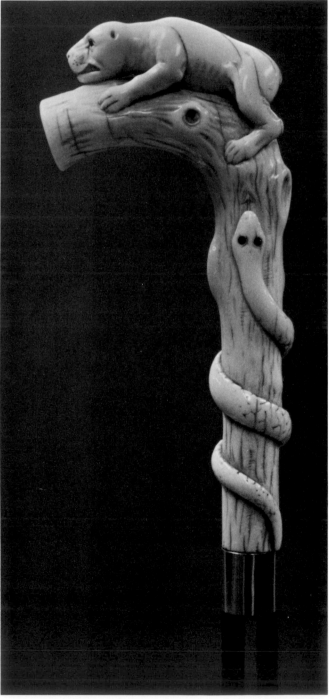

230 A snake curling around its own body, head down. Unusual European ivory carving. By tradition, sticks with snakes facing downwards were preferably worn by pharmacists. Probably turn of the 20th century. Height 16 cm.

228 The serpent's head is set with rubies as eyes, the silver is green and blue enamelled and chased with floral decoration. The unusual handle is heart shaped. Lady's cane from the Art Nouveau period. Probably an umbrella handle rather than cane handle. Height 15 cm.

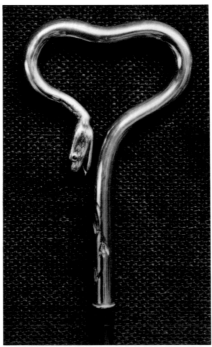

228 △   229 ▽

229 A snake is curling around the yellow patinated ivory handle, the knob of which is decorated with carved snakes' heads and set with a dark green serpentine (as protection against snake bites). The shaft is also ivory. Probably Indian, 19th century.

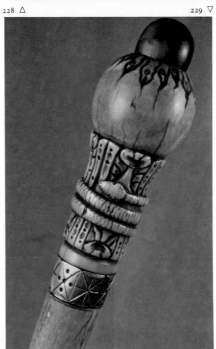

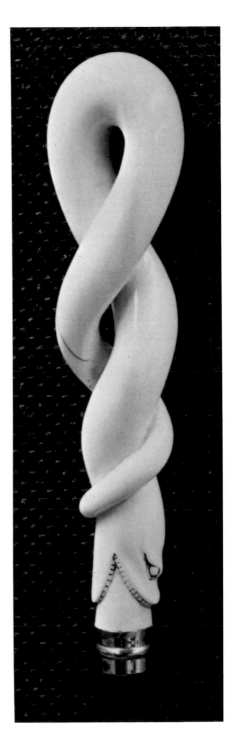

231 Ornaments and images are colored straw glued to the surface. Executed by a prisoner of war during the Napoleonic period. Very rare. Overall length 92 cm.

232 Multi-color gold and lacquer relief is called "Takamakie." Umbrella and cane handles by the Japanese master Kumei. Height 21,5 cm.

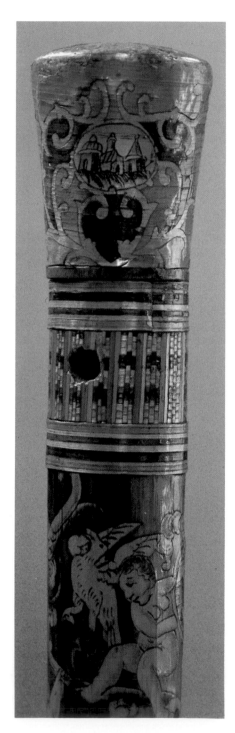

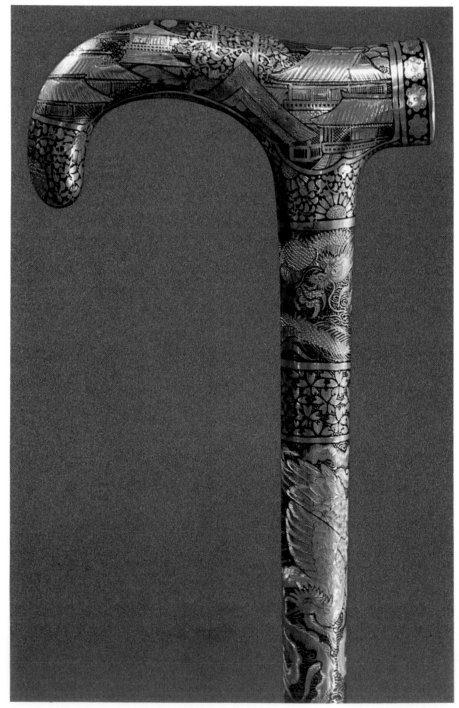

233 *Mother of pearl cranes, gold leaves, lacquered birds laid in ivory by the Japanese artist's dynasty Shibayama. The technique is named after this family. Precious knob (circa 1800). Height 8 cm.*

234 *A silver Tako, the octopus in Japanese mythology, is sitting in an ivory handle. Height 10 cm.*

235 *A metal lobster is sitting on a piece of knotty wood. A real shell was electroplated. Japanese piece, early 20th century.*

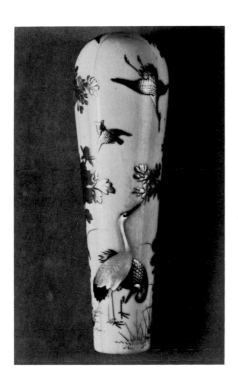

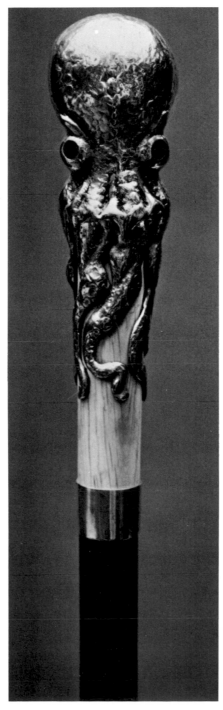

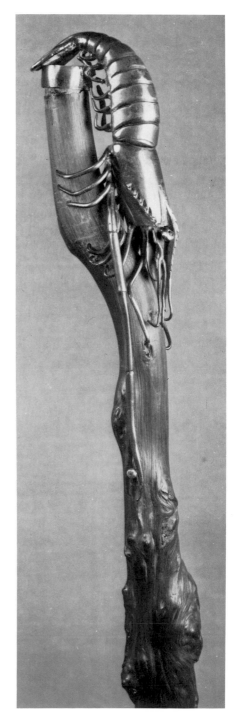

236 *A horse's head with saddle as handle, bearing the Greek inscription "Kerkyra," with or without a male bearded face on the opposite side, was the typical souvenir from Korfu from the turn of the 20th century.*

237 *Elephant's head carved from ebony wood with ivory tusks and bold carving at the shaft. Typical souvenir from Ceylon, circa 1900. Length of handle 12.5 cm.*

238 *Shepherd's crook from Scotland with "Neck Crook" and stylized thistle end. Contemporary all wood cane.*

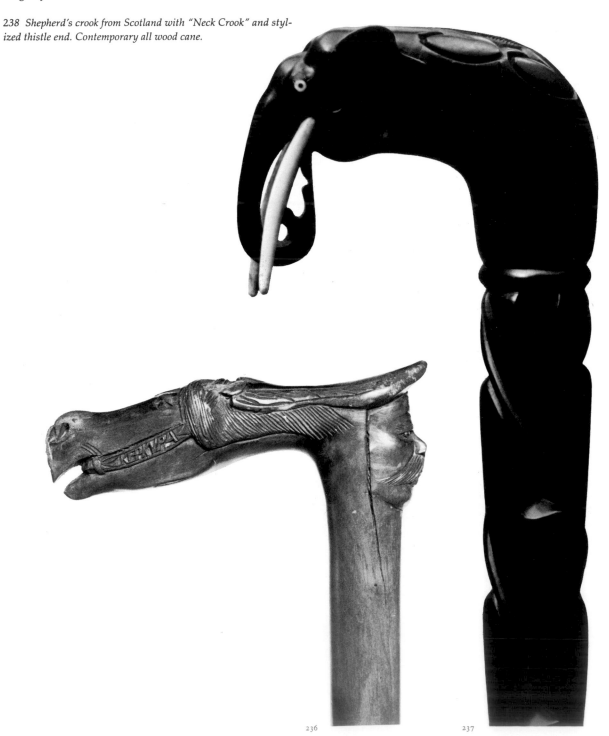

236   237   238

239 *"Le Makila" from the Basque lands. The stick with an iron ring, lead filling and soldered coin. The knob handle is horn and can be unscrewed and reveals a metal pin (Pique). Made to date by J. Leoncini.*

240 *Cane made of shark's spine from the Seychelles islands and cane sword "Gupti" from India with bone inlay. Careless and badly executed contemporary souvenirs.*

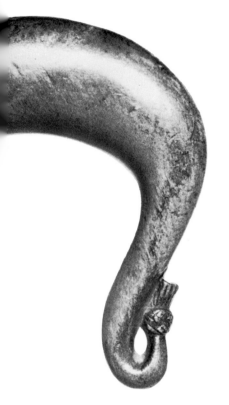

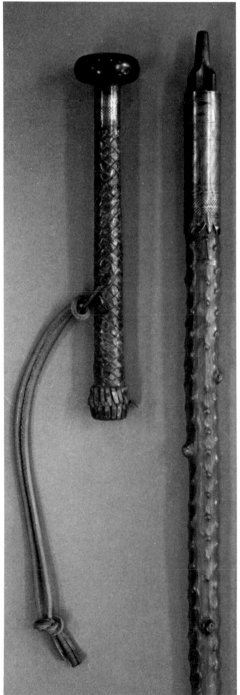

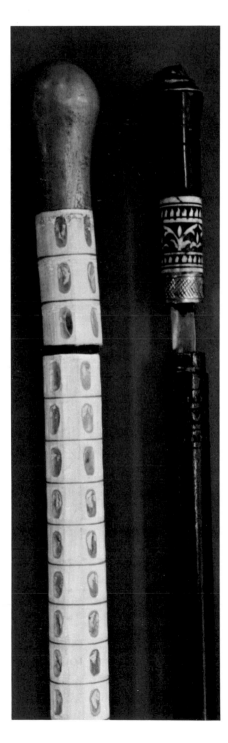

241 *Whiskey gauge ivory knob. 1/16 Gill = 1 cl for the drink on the road.*

242 *The cork screw with horn handle is screwed into the shaft. Circa 1890.*

243 *The wooden fist contains a nut cracker, which is operated with a screw.*

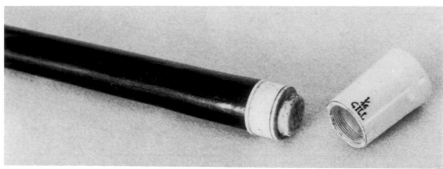

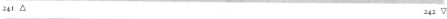

241 △

242 ▽

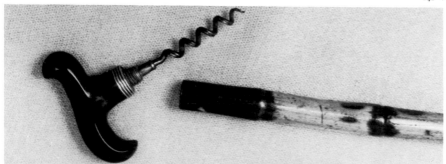

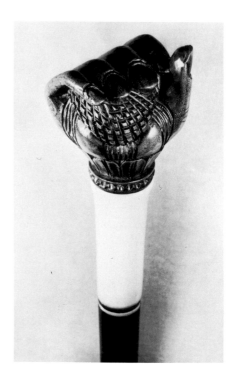

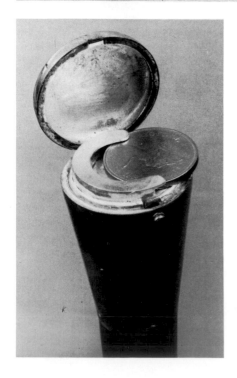

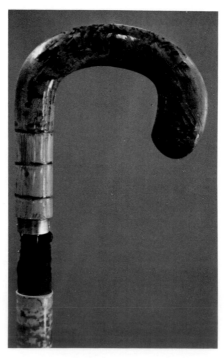

244 *The silver pennies for the coach are at the gentleman's fingertip. These portemonnais are usually very well executed.*

245 *Simple umbrella case: The umbrella is attached to the handle. The shaft can be folded like a telescope and put in the pocket.*

246 The umbrella silk table is stretched over four sticks, which, together with the legs and the fabric, are contained in the upper part of the case, which can be unscrewed from the handle. English patent from 1891.

247 The silver conical shaped handle contains nutmeg and a grater, the lower portion is a pepper dispenser. English, late 19th century.

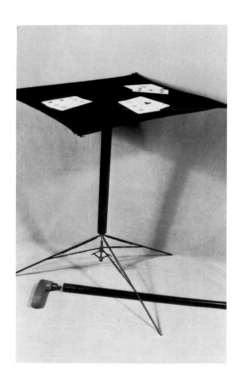

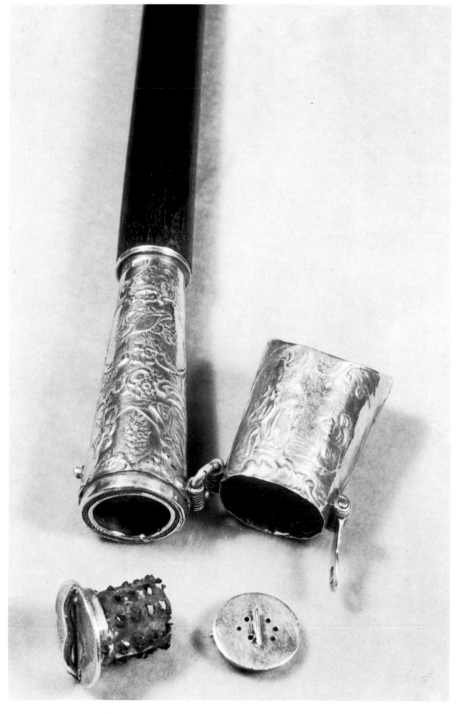

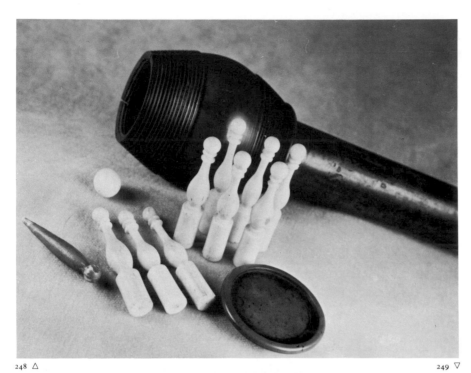

248 *A wooden barrel shaped handle contains a table bowling set. Ball and skittle are made of ivory. Middle 19th century.*

248 △   249 ▽

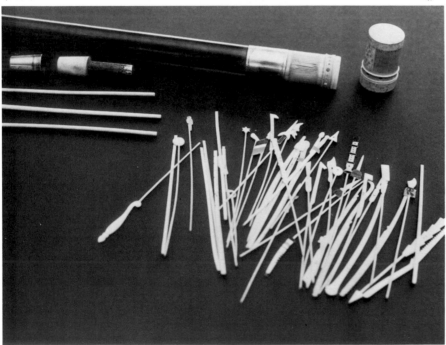

249 *Spillikin game. Made by French prisoner's of war from whale bones during the Napoleonic wars. (circa 1810).*

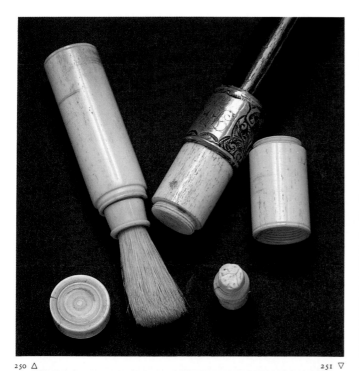

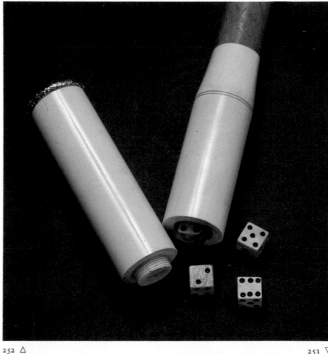

250 △   251 ▽   252 △   253 ▽

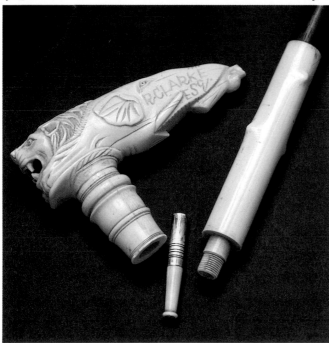

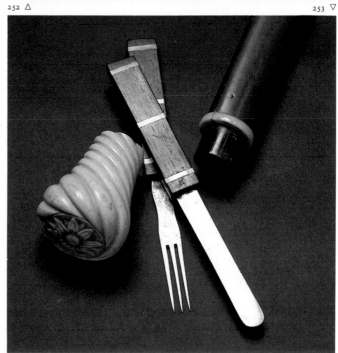

250 The long, straight ivory handle can be unscrewed and contains
shaving soap, set in ivory, a shaving brush and a small container for
water to beat the foam. The silver band is engraved, inscribed and
dated 1895.

251 Three part ivory handle, Carved handle with stylized lions and
elephant heads. Boldly inscribed "R. Clarke Esq." Turned middle piece,
which can be unscrewed and contains as opium needle. Overall height
18 cm.

252 The long massive ivory straight handle (Height 19 cm) has a
gilded plate and is mounted on malacca cane. Can be opened to reveal
4 dice, the ivory piece on the cane may be used as a dice box. Circa
1890.

253 Turned ivory handle with carved Edelweiss mounted on a heavy
malacca shaft with ebony ferrule and iron nail. The cane contains a
folded knife and fork with metal set wooden handles. Inscription on
the blade "W.H. Wragg's patent." Size of silverware 18 cm.

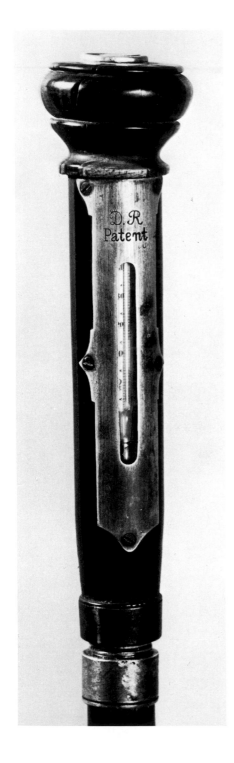
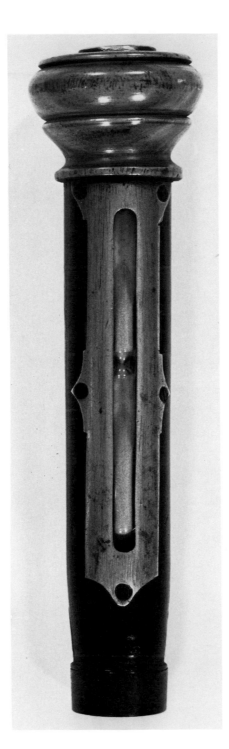

254, 255 *The knob contains a compass, thermometer and 5 minute hour-glass on each side of the handle which can be unscrewed. The shaft holds a container with ether to kill insects. The lower portion of the shaft has a 50 cm surveyor's rod with 1 and 10 cm calibrations. A gardener's knife unfolds at the ferrule. German patent from November 1877.*

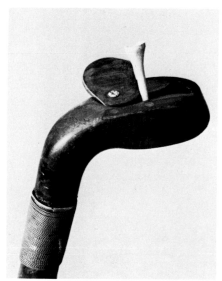

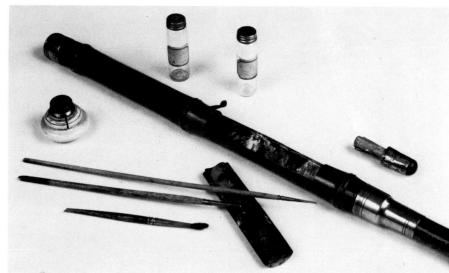

256 △   257 ▽ 258 △   259 ▽

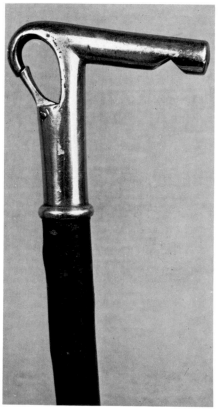

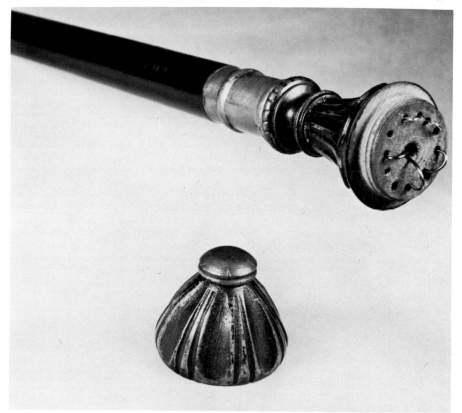

256 Walking cane in the form of a golf club, the handle containing the tee. Allows for practice during the walk.

257 Spring hook for dog leash or collar. The handle contains a dog whistle. Nickeled iron.

258 Painter's cane with ivory knob. The knob containing the kerosene burner and two containers for liquids. The middle part can be opened and holds pigment pots, the removed lid is the palette. The brushes are held by the ferrule. Last third 19th century.

259 The metal knob will safely store fishing hooks. The shaft contains the pole.

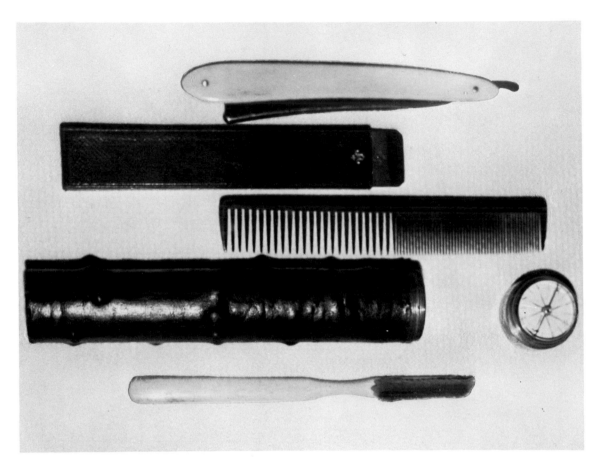

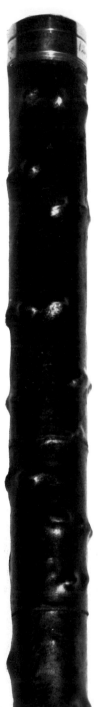

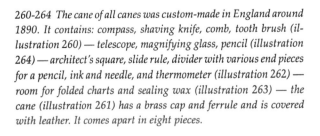

260-264 *The cane of all canes was custom-made in England around 1890. It contains: compass, shaving knife, comb, tooth brush (illustration 260) — telescope, magnifying glass, pencil (illustration 264) — architect's square, slide rule, divider with various end pieces for a pencil, ink and needle, and thermometer (illustration 262) — room for folded charts and sealing wax (illustration 263) — the cane (illustration 261) has a brass cap and ferrule and is covered with leather. It comes apart in eight pieces.*

261

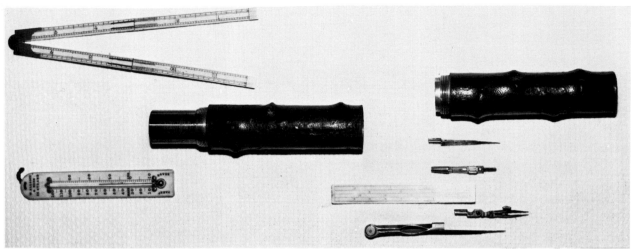

262 △

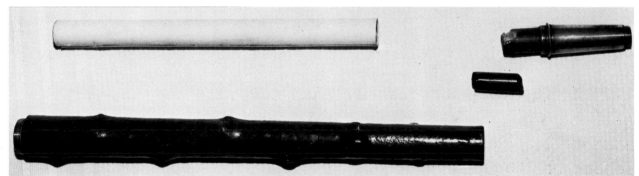

263 △   264 ▽

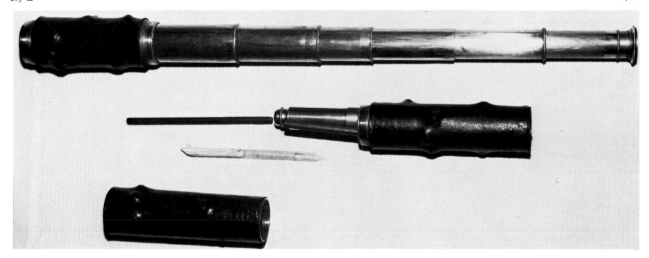

265   *Silver cigarette holder in the form of an Indian's head. The ivory hat forms the mouth piece. Length 8 cm.*

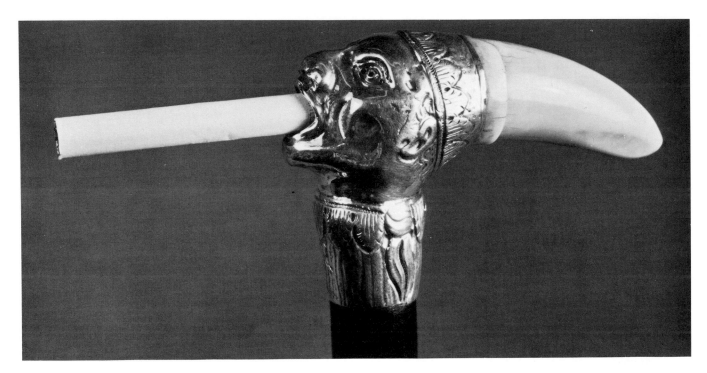

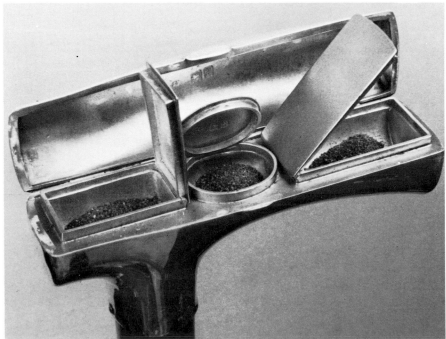

266 *Silver snuff box with two compartments. A mixing bowl in the middle. The tight fitting lids well executed. England, 1896.*

267 Metal cigar cutter. A functional rather than beautiful handle.

268 The front section of the deer's antler can be opened and contains a basin for snuffing in silver. Heavily chased, wide silver band, London marks 1904.

269 The silvered metal handle contains a gas lighter. Quite a common model from 1920.

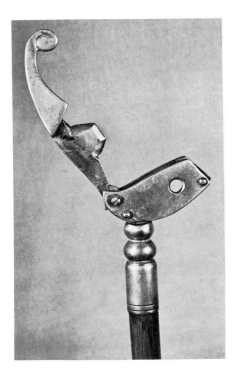

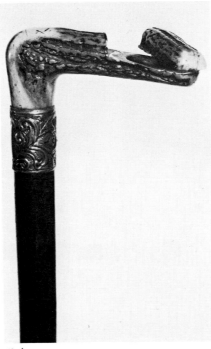

268 △

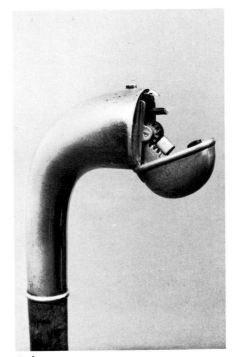

269 △

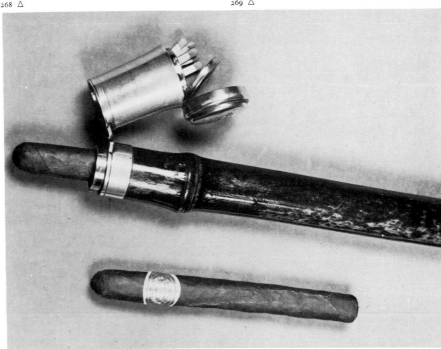

270 The shafts holds two cigars, the silver knob holds the matches. The inner lid has a rubbing surface.

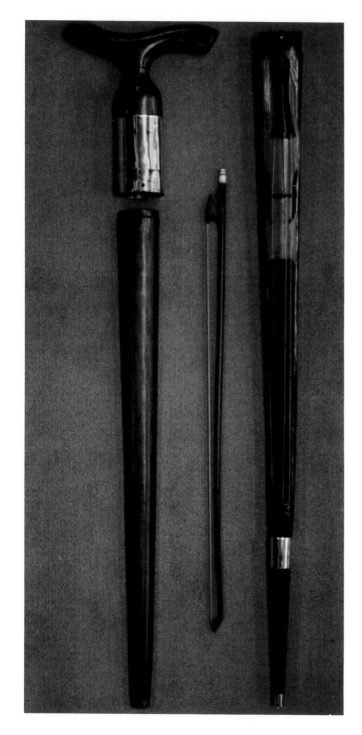

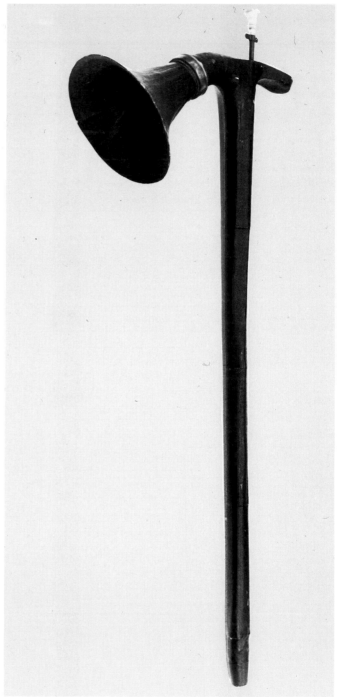

271 Opened violin cane. The removed cover plate and ebony handle, which is again attached to the sounding board as a chin piece. When folded, the bow is hidden. Soft, light wood, probably pine, brass fitting monogrammed "A.A.," circa 1800. Length 89 cm.

272 Horn cane, the mouth and tube pieces are contained in the handle. The tube set in the shaft has double cane length. 19th century. Paris, Musee de Conservatoire National de Musique

273 Cane clarinet made from imitation bamboo with twelve wooden keys, set into the bamboo rings. 19th Century. Height 89 cm.
Berlin, Museum of Musical Instruments of the Federal Institute for Musical Research.
(Berlin, Musikinstrumenten-Museum des Staatl. Institutes fur Musikforschung)

274 Flageolet with brass key. Animal handle. These nozzle flutes have a sharper sound than their relatives the recorder flutes. 19th Century. Height 89 cm.
Berlin, Museum for Musical Instruments of the Federal Institute for Musical Research (Berlin, Musikinstrumenten-Museum des Staatl. Institutes fur Musikforschung)

275 German flute cane. Ivory knob and ferrule, hole for band attachment. Four brass keys. Middle 19th century. Height 90 cm.
Berlin, Museum for Musical Instruments of the Federal Institute for Musical Research (Berlin, Musikinstrumenten-Museum des Staatl. Institutes fur Musikforschung)

276 German flute and clarinet in one cane, mouth piece in the handle. Clarinet in F with five wooden keys, German flute in E minor with one key. In addition, the shaft is brand marked with a measure calibrated for an old German unit. From the atelier of Ulrich Amann in the Toggenburg area (Germany), circa 1810. Height 90 cm.
Nuernberg, Germanic National Museum

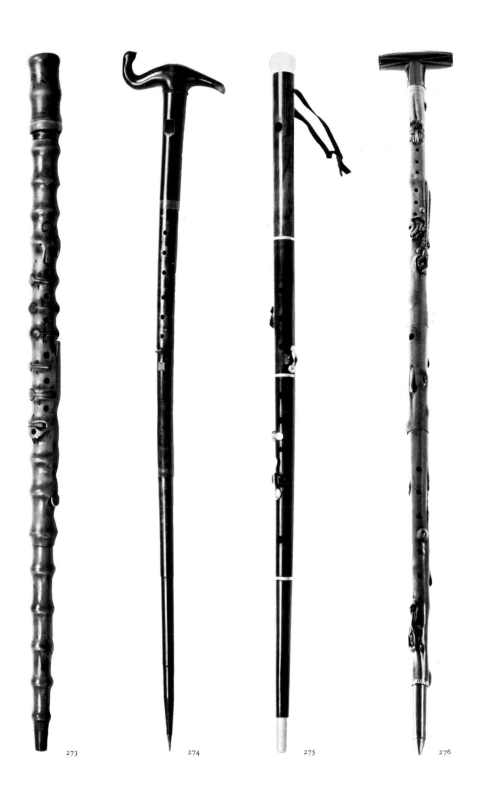

273   274   275   276

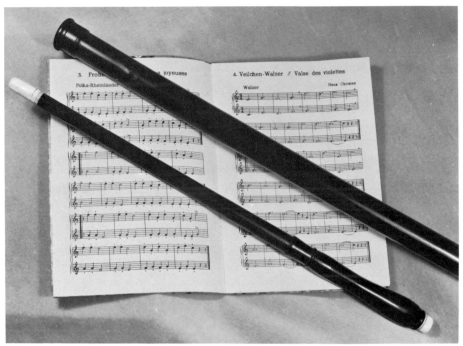

277 German flute with ivory end pieces, which is hidden in a polished wooden cane. Height 90 cm.

278 Czakan harmonica with cover, which is used as rhythmic instrument. This cane instrument in axe form is a traditional Hungarian souvenir.

279 Hearing aid as walking stick. A model by Frank Valery, Paris, which was shown at the world exhibition in Amsterdam in 1909 and received a silver medal. A rare collector's item.

277 △   278 ▽

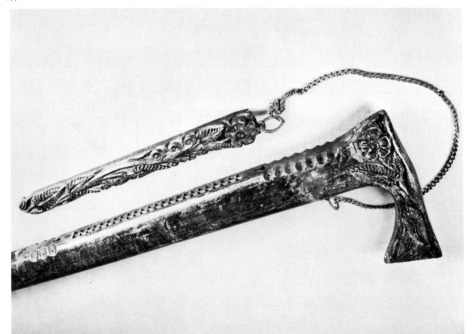

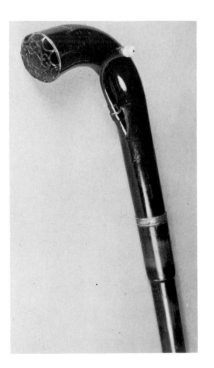

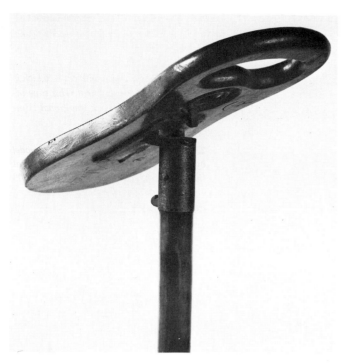

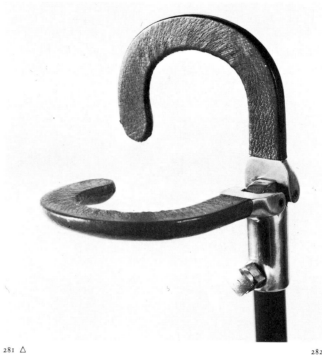

281 △

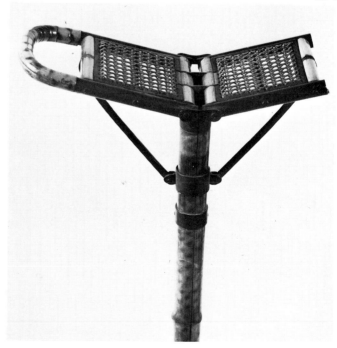

282 ▽

280-282 The sitting and shooting cane was invented in England around 1813. Since then there have been 300 different patents and many more models for such canes. The wooden cane (illustration 280) and the reeded cane (illustration 282) are from the turn of the century. The leather covered aluminum cane is a contemporary example (illustration 281). Their most important quality is that folded they have to be good walking and support sticks.

283 *Metal cane, imitating wood, the wooden knob can be removed and contains measuring cups with 4 different scales and the inscriptions "Beer Gallons" and "Wine Gallons." The measuring stick has a brass handle and tip. The cane has a 12 cm long ferrule and is very heavy.*

284 *The "Calculator" is a forerunner of the computer. It could be used to multiply, divide and calculate the angle. It was used during the First World War be English officers.*

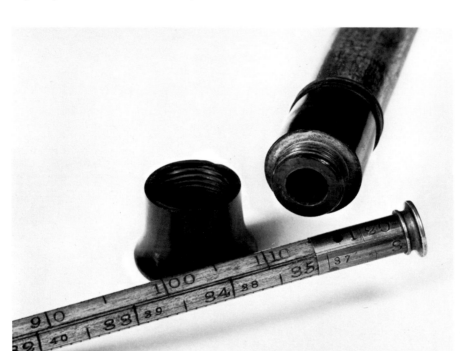

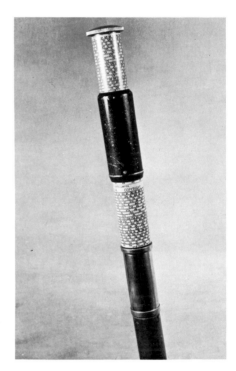

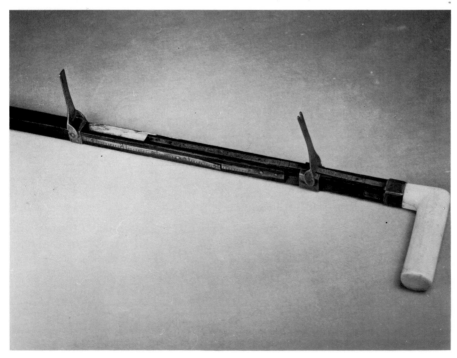

285 *Shoemaker's cane in tetragonal wood with an ivory handle. The various bars, which unfold and slide, are made of brass to measure the foot size. The same gauge, however, not attached to a cane, is currently in use by English shoemakers. Turn of the 20th century.*

286 Coffin maker's cane, which can be extended sufficiently to discreetly measure the length of a corpse.

287 Step calculator or Pedometer, signed "Sisson. Invet. London." Does not count the number of steps made, but rather the distance passed. The large hand can measure up to 40 calibrations, the small one 32. One increment of the large hand is 1 rod = 5.02 meters, 40 rod = 1/8 of a mile. When the little hand turns once around the dial, a 4 mile distance has been walked. Circa 1730.

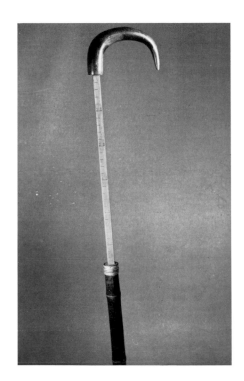

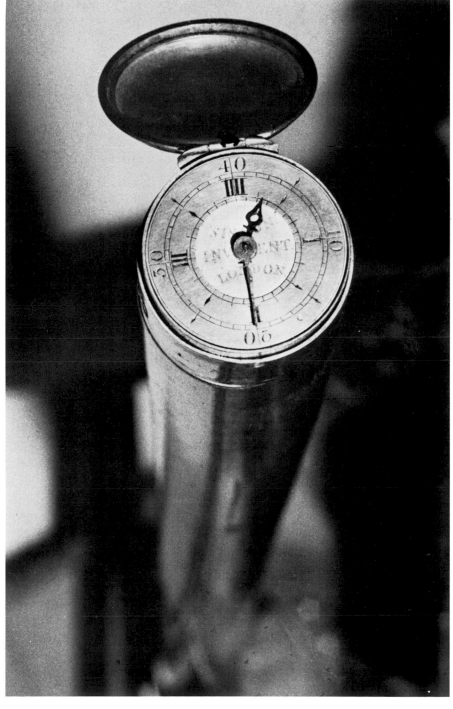

288 Monocle set on an elegantly slim ebony cane, to see at a distance in the Opera or as a loupe. The lens is embedded in a crystal ring. France, circa 1900.

289 Opera binoculars, which are held by a silver hand. 19th Century

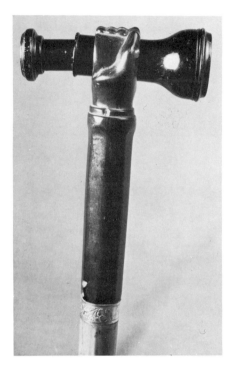

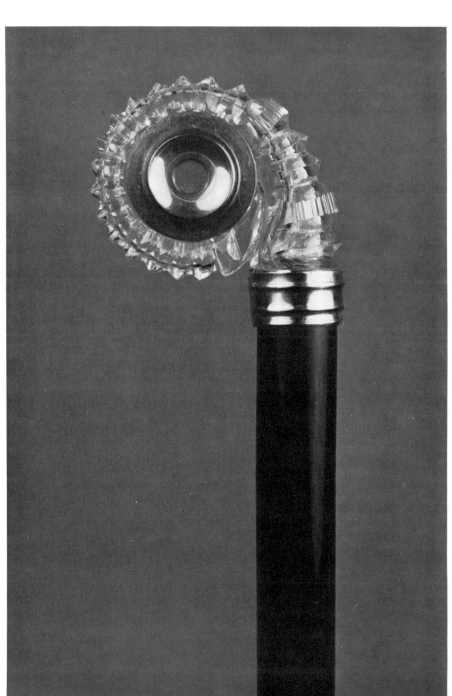

290 Cane with silver set knob, containing a glass case. Cane
and glasses were made for each other and the style of glasses
dates the set as early Biedermeier.

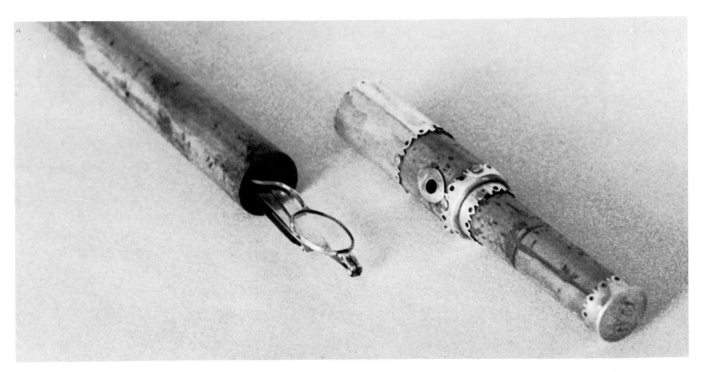

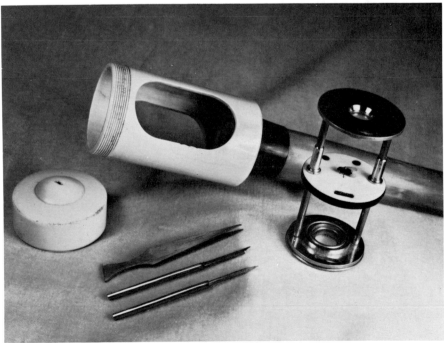

291 The ivory handle unscrews and contains
a strong loupe and a viewing plate. The instrument has two different lenses. Additions
include tweezers and 2 other instruments.
Probably custom-made.

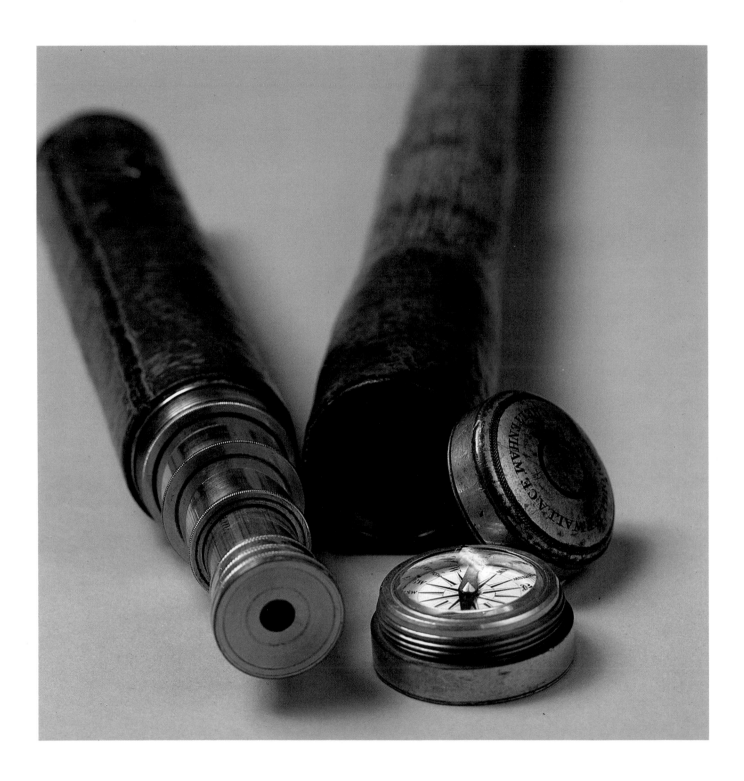

292 *Heavy bamboo cane, the upper third is leather covered. Two brass caps can be unscrewed and brass rimmed rings for carrying bands. Inscription on the cap "H.P. Wallace. Priory Lodge Cheltenham." Contains a compass and a triple folding telescope, fully extended 43 cm long, with the owner's inscription "Abraham Bath." Circa 1850.*

293, 294   *The Cane Camera "Ben Akiba" (illustration 193, closed) was invented by Emil Kronke, Dresden (German Patent 143.649 from February 26, 1902) and manufactured by A. Lehmann, Berlin, circa 1903. The photographs had a size of 1.3 x 2.5 cm on a roll of film 1.8 cm wide, allowing for 20 photos. The lens (f= 1:9/35 mm) aimed through the short end of the handle. The long side of the handle contained 4 additional rolls of film.*

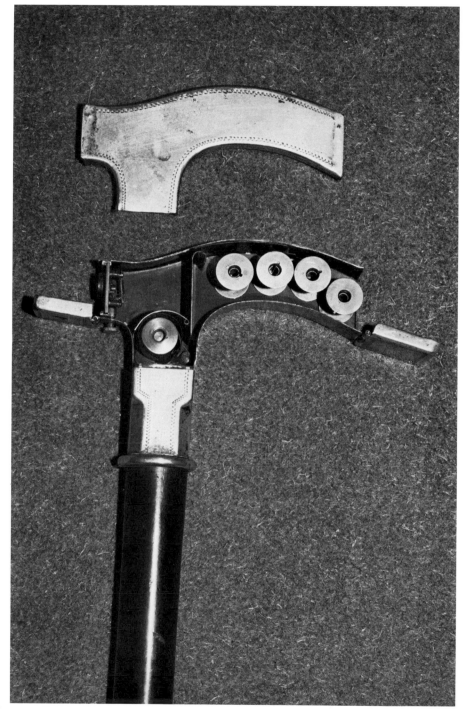

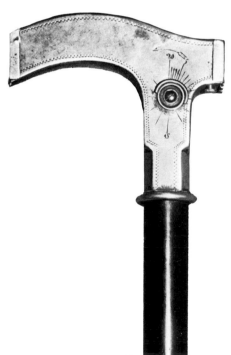

293   294

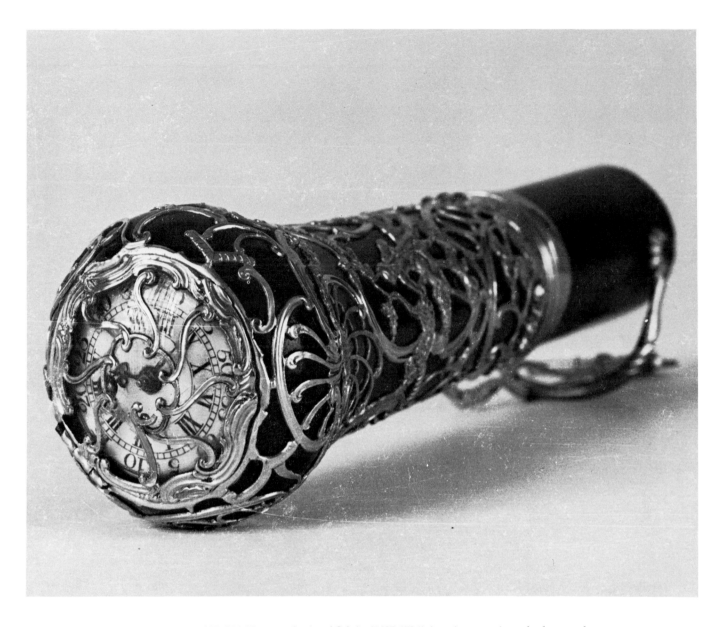

295, 296 Verge watch, signed Cabrier (1697-1724), is set in a green jasper knob, covered with gold filigree decoration. Formerly owned by Kurfuerst Maximilian III. Joseph of Bavaria. Illustration 296 shows the side view.
Munich, Nymphenburg castle.

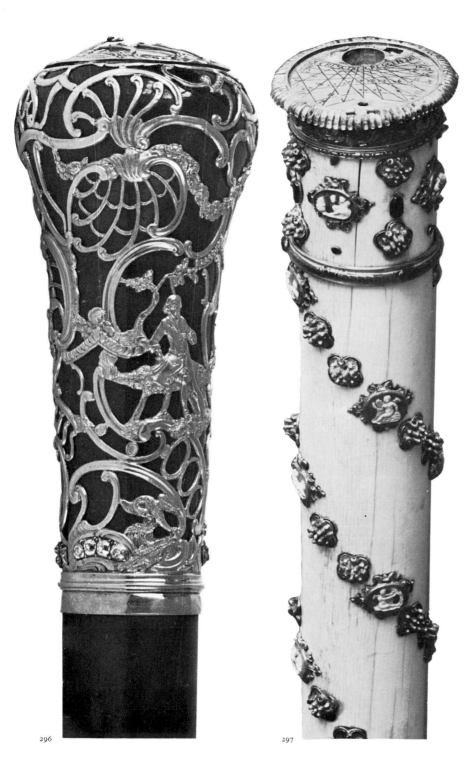

297 *Sun dial cane, owned by Duke Albrecht V of Bavaria (1550-1579), the first time described in an inventory listing in 1598. The cane is made from one piece of ivory, length 150 cm and diameter 2.5 cm, the sundial and the three tipped ferrule are gold. The cane is decorated with a string of gold nails, cabochon gem stones and framed cameos from Italy. The cane was made by either Abraham Lotter or Ulrich Eberl. The gnomon could be folded before closing the lid. The gnomon, the gem stone covered lid and a compass are missing. Munich, Nymphenburg castle.*

296

297

298, 299, 301 *In 1885, a long baguette movement (illustration 298, 299) was patented for L. Holuska to be used exclusively for watch canes. It is wound by the handle or knob. The dial is on the side of the shaft and rather small and behind thick glass to protect it against shock should the cane fall. The ball form knob (illustration 301) bears unidentifiable silver marks. This cane contains movement from illustration 298, 299.*

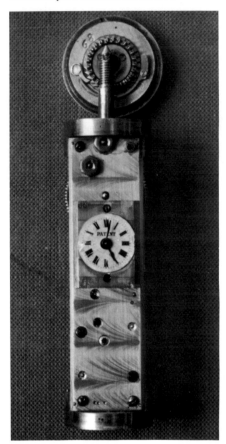

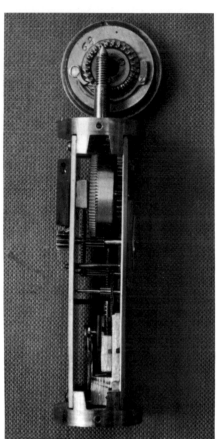

299 △

300 ▽

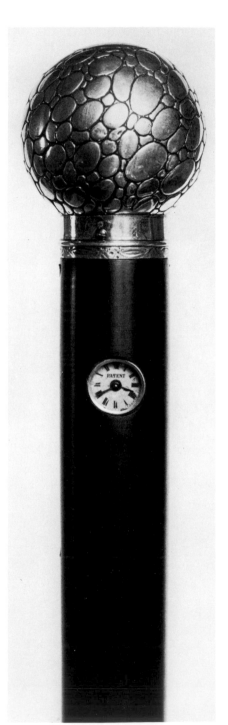

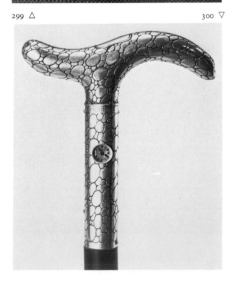

300 *The Fritskrucke is signed "M. Halbkram, Vienna, Kaertnerstr. 20." Diameter of dial 1 cm. Frequently the cane has been cut at the shaft below the dial.*

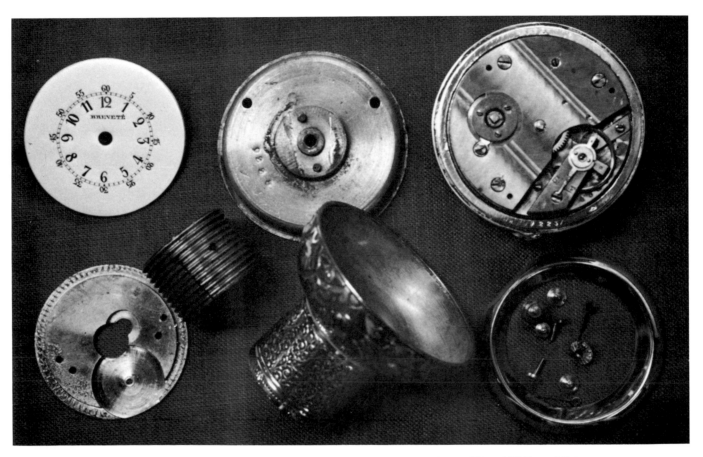

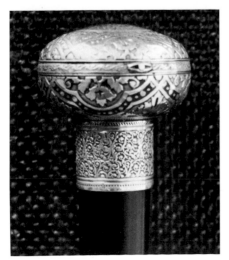

302, 303 Walking case with silver and enamel hinged lid. Enamel dial with arabic numerals, Swiss patent, silver content 900 and 2 Swiss hallmarks. The hands are set by the crown, which attaches to the hands through the crystal. The watch is wound by turning the knob of the cane. Height of knob with lid 4 cm.

304 *The dial is decorated with a multi-color rural scene painted in a provincial style, the lid is embossed with a mountain flower. Winding crown on the side, a Swiss patent from 1899. Diameter 6.5 cm.*

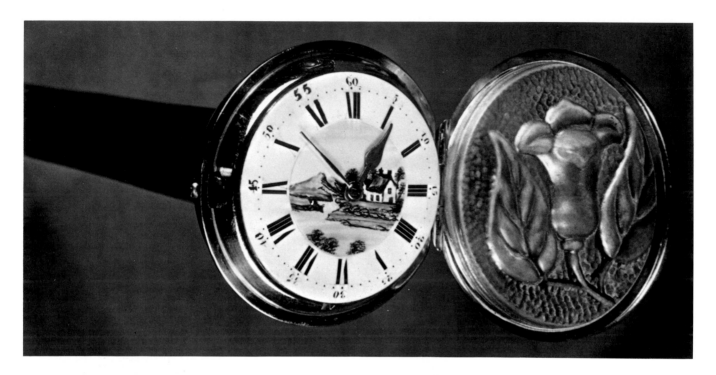

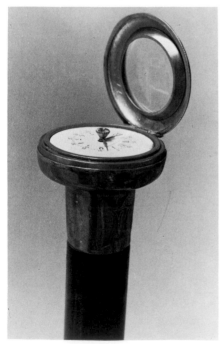

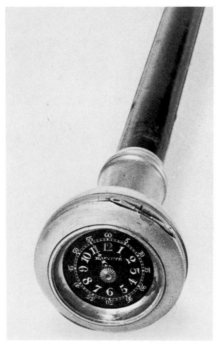

305 *Walking cane watch, Swiss patent from 1888, turning of bezel winds the watch, setting crown for hands on dial. Silver and gold with monogram and London hallmarks, 1894.*

306 *Watch cane (similar to illustration 305) with black dial and inscribed Breveté (patented). Circa 1900. Diameter 4 cm.*

307, 308 An ivory ball is inscribed as a globe. The example on the left shows ships and whales inhabiting the oceans. The one on the right can be opened to reveal a sun dial. Scrimshaw from the 19th century. Both mounted on malacca cane. Diameter of globe 5 cm.

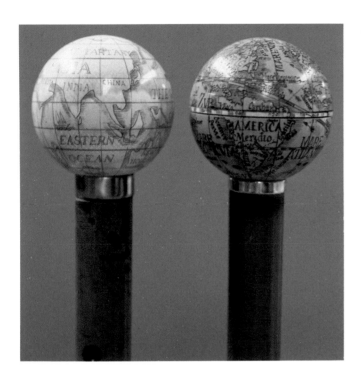

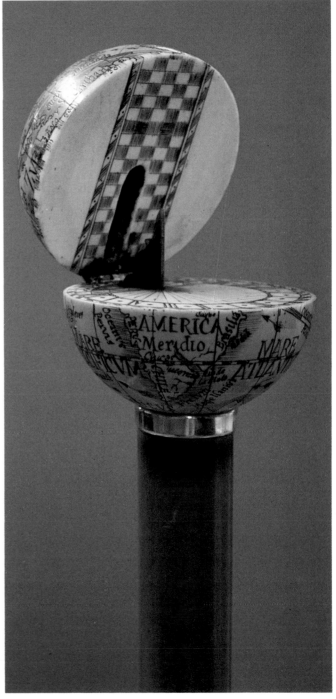

309 *A flint-lock pistol and a sword are set in a cane. The pistol is inscribed "Kleft Inventor" on one side and "London" on the other. H.W. Van der Kleft obtained several patents around 1810 for various cane system combinations.*

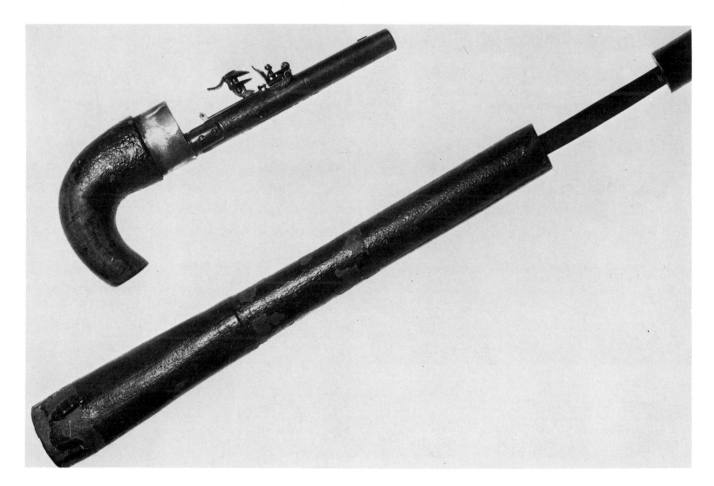

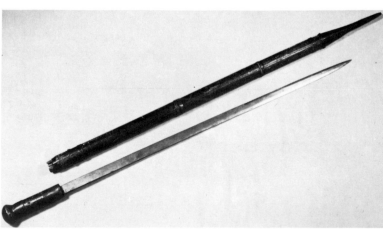

310 *This rather insignificant but fairly aged cane is covered with leather. Probably 17th Century.*

311 *Air gun as walking cane made of black leather covered iron with ivory knob and brass ferrule. With air pump to fill the air chamber (middle). 400 pumps will create pressure for 20 shots. On the right the barrel with notch and bead sights, and release button on the side. Was loaded from the front. Weight 3.5 kg. England, circa 1850. (see also illustration 41).*

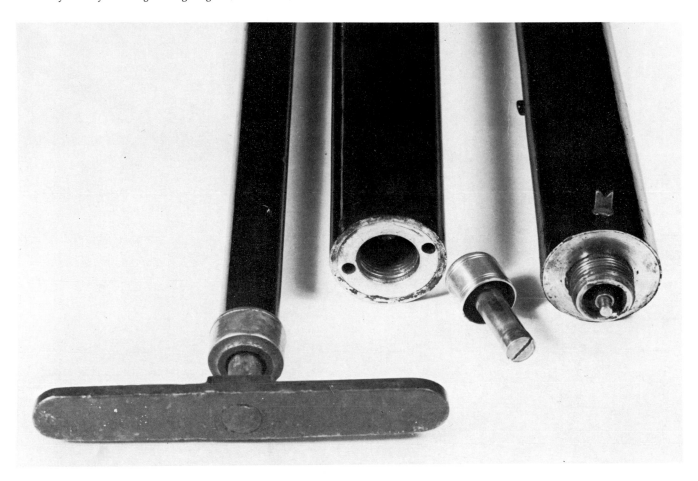

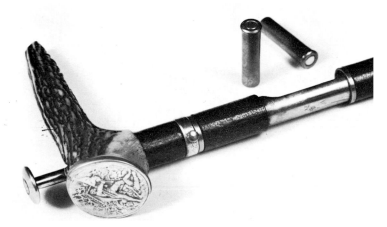

312 *Iron, leather covered shot gun with deer antler handle, the rose covered by embossed silver medal, showing the Blacksmith of Kochel in battle. The gun was made for 9 mm caliber with No. 8 lead. The shot gun is set in the illustration.*

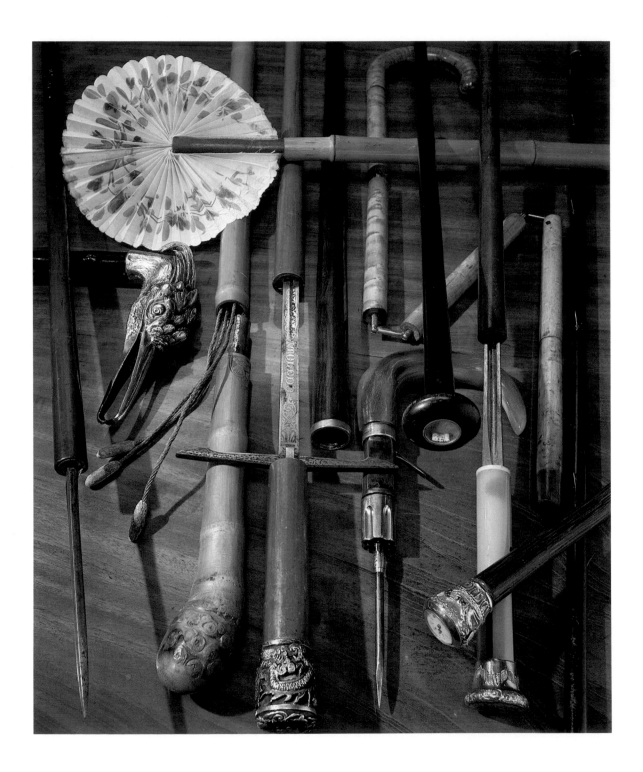

313 This composition of selected system canes shows from left to right: cane, which can release a sword blade, heavy bird's head with pointed beak, a perfect weapon cane containing a three weighted flails, a Toledo sword cane with extending hand guard, pepper box pistol with center spike, a traveling cane folding into three pieces, a gambler's cane with dice in the handle, a cane with a triangular gouge blade to check the contents of a tub or sack to make sure the contents are as advertised all the way through, a weapons cane with metal spikes extending from the shaft, and a fan cane for a lady.

314, 315 Ivory knight with full armor, coat, helmet with feathers and lifted shield, carved with armorial crest and a fraternity emblem in the middle. Exceptional student cane from the Teutonia fraternity, Jena. Height 15 cm.

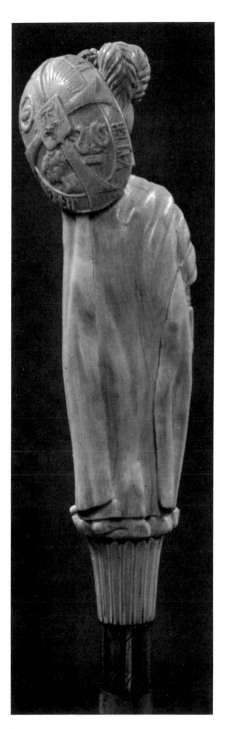
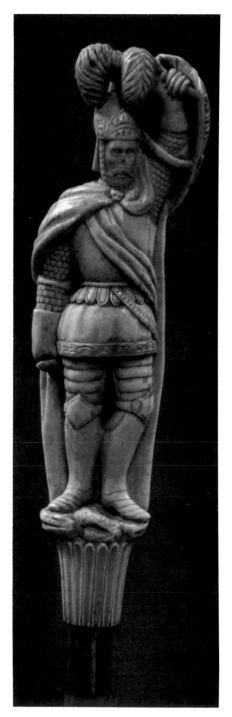

316, 317 *The short ivory handle widens at the end and bears a finely carved family crest. The front bears the fraternity emblem of the Frankonia, Hannover (?), in raised relief. Shaft made of malacca cane. Ivory ferrule. Height of handle 11 cm.*

318 *Large pistol shaped ivory cane handle, with rich armorial crest, fraternity emblem of the Helvetia, Zurich and dated 15. II. 1878. Probably made by Glaser & Son, Dresden.*

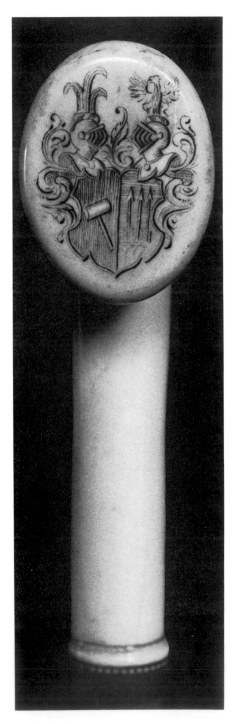

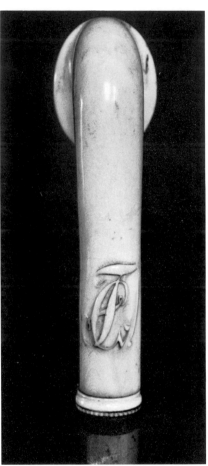

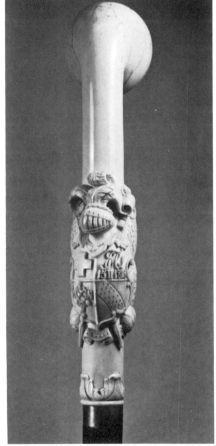

◁ 316   317 △   318 △

319 Large Armorial crest on a pistol shaped ivory handle (detail) with fraternity emblem of Corps Saxonia, Hannover.

320 The front of an ivory handle carved with a fraternity emblem in high relief (enlarged illustration). Fraternity Arminia a.d. Burgkeller, Jena. End 19th Century.

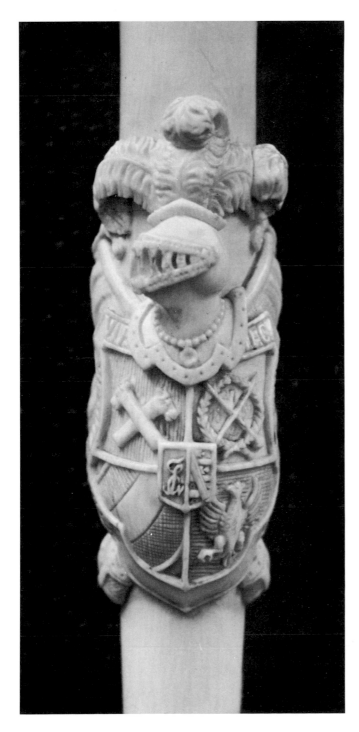

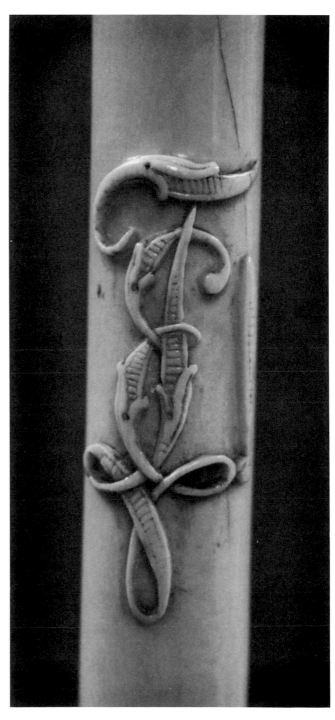

321 *Wooden ax cane of a Hungarian shepherd, inlaid with brass threads and nails, decorated with red and blue pearls. Too well executed for a souvenir piece.*

322 *Well carved handle made from walrus in two parts. A miner with a light and ax is carved from the tooth. In the romantic style around 1850.*

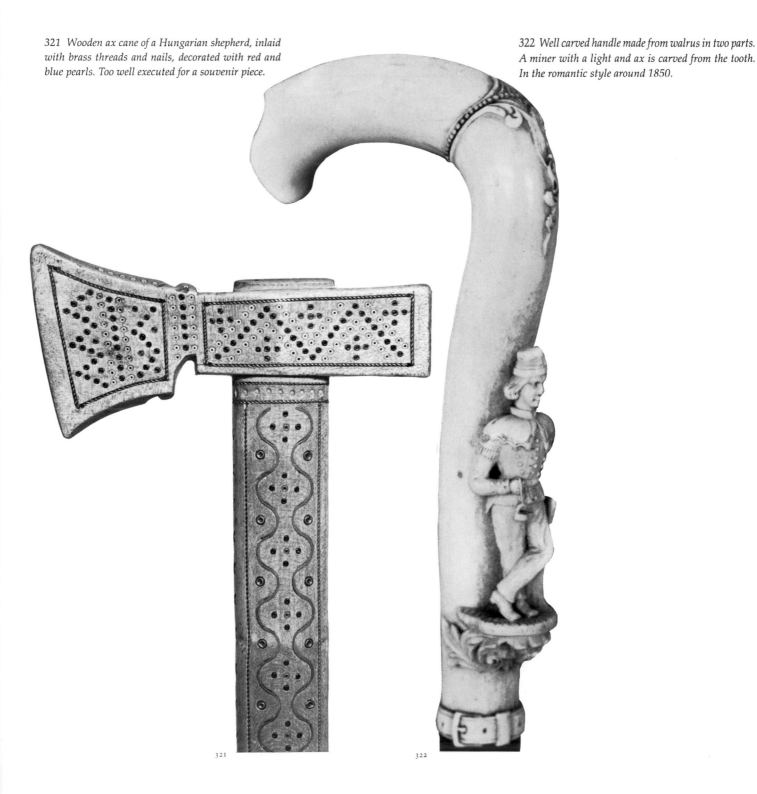

321   322

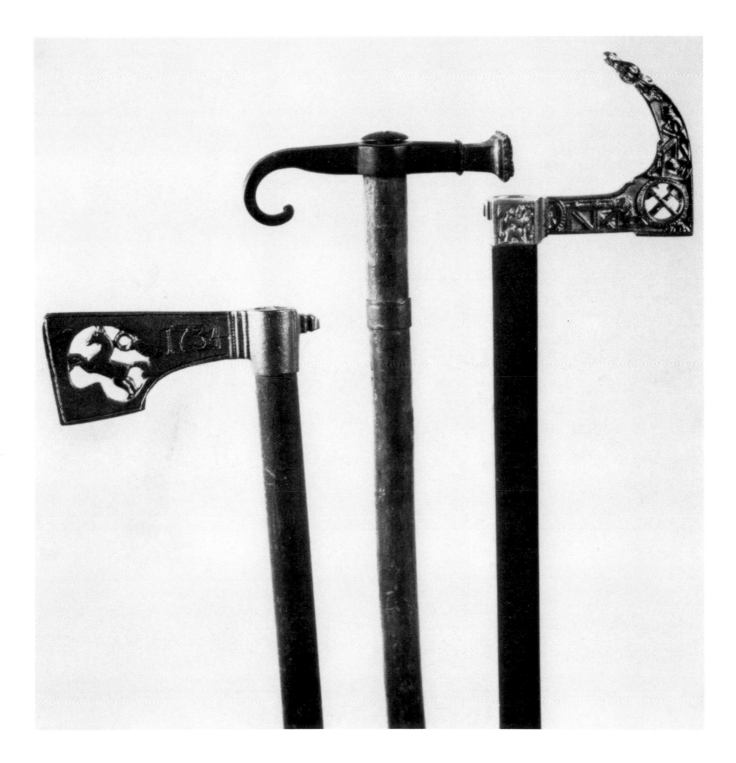

323 *From left to right: Presentation ax cane from Lower Saxonia. Recast of an old model, still presented. — Antique utility cane, which used to be carried by officials, never by simple workers. The tip was curved to secure the lamp. — Recast of an old presentation cane in brass form Peisenberg.*

324, 325 *Ivory head, the various areas of the brain engraved on the skull and the corresponding spiritual and physical characteristics inscribed on the bust. Diagnostic cane for followers of the Gallic Skull theory. England, early 19th century. Height 6.2 cm.*

326 *Knob can be unscrewed, with pierced lid. Decorated with silver nails in pique pattern. Malacca shaft with hole for carrying band. The compartment of this cane houses either smelling salts or sponges with vinegar. Typical doctor's cane from England. 1st half 18th*

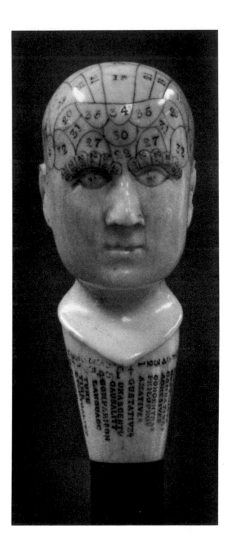

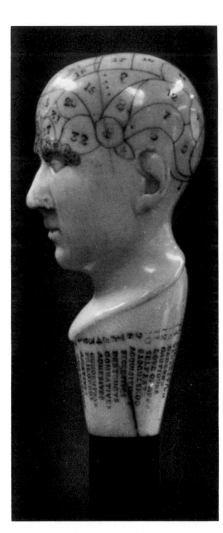

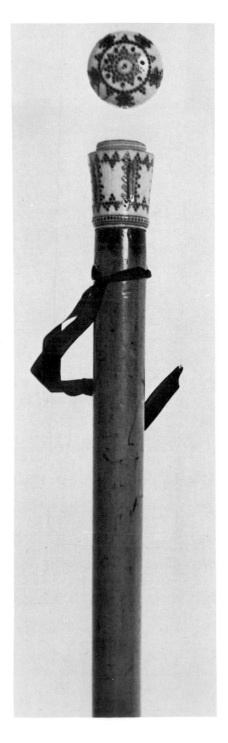

327, 328 *Both canes have long ivory handles in classical form, the one on the right the pistol shaped handle — Partial view (illustration 327): The raised relief carving on the left shows two horses and three dogs, the one on the right, with darker patina, shows three horses and one dog. Both also show the rider's utensils. Lovingly and artistically executed pieces from the Saxonian region, similar, but not made by the same artist. 2nd half 19th century, Height 17 and 19 cm.*

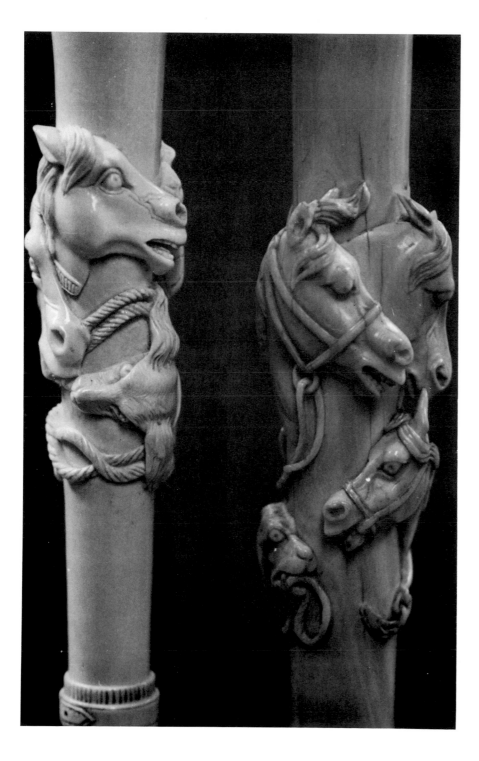

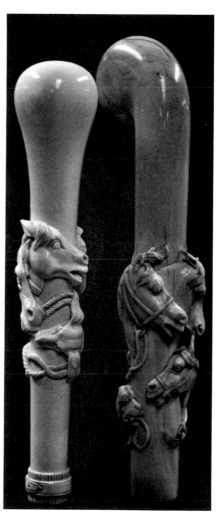

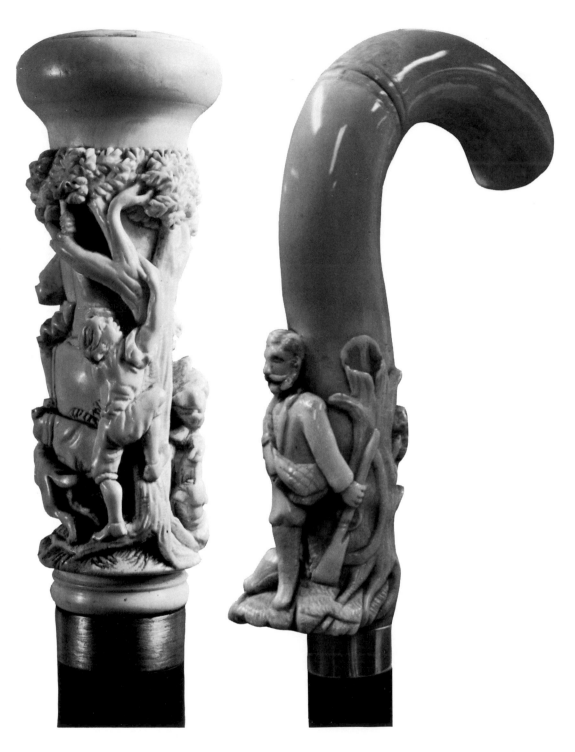

329 *The knob with exceptionally fine and rich ivory relief carving. Hunting scene with dog, wild boar, tree and hunter.*

330 *Handle in two parts carved from walrus tooth, decorated with hunter, standing on top of his prey. Dresden or Bautzen. Middle of 19th century. Height 12 cm.*

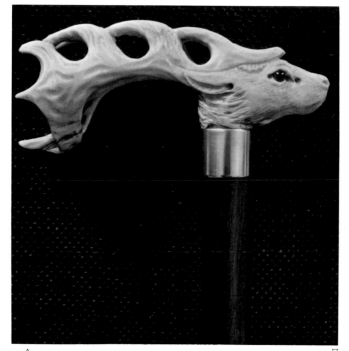

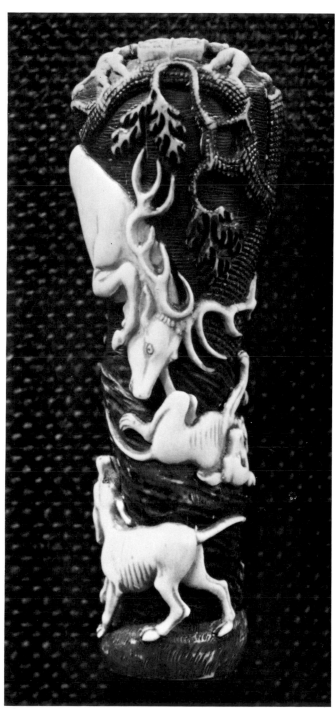

331 △   332 ▽

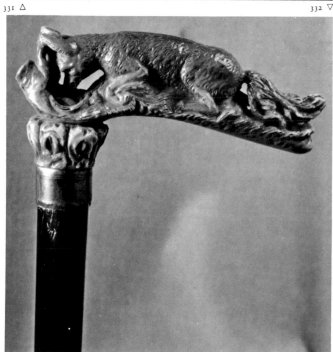

331 *Unusual ivory handle, deer head and antlers, filigree carved in one tooth. Probably 19th century, provenance unknown.*

332 *The fox, sniffing in a den, is carved stained ivory. The bottom plate and back of fox make this a walking cane, which fits well into the hand.*

333 *Deer fighting with attacking dogs. Magnificent ivory handle. The knob is also engraved with armorial crest. The decor is heightened by the partial coloration of the ivory. Geislingen (?). Height 14 cm.*

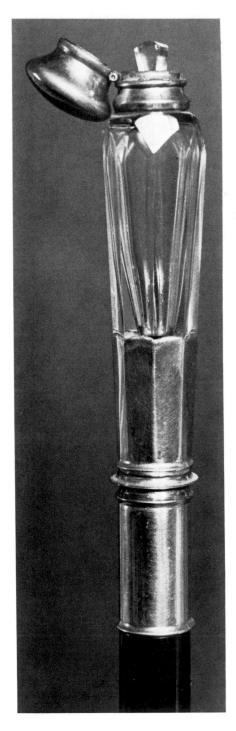

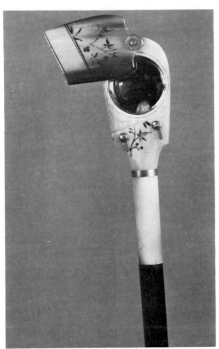

334 Crystal bottle with glass stopper and gilded cover lid, used as perfume bottle. Mounted on black lacquered shaft. The ring is hallmarked "DO 18 ct G.P." (Gold plated). England, circa 1914. Height of bottle 14 cm.

335 Horn handle painted with flowers, which can be opened o reveal a small mirror. lady's cane from the turn of the twentieth century. Diameter of mirror 4 cm.

336 Horn handle with metal band. In the upper third of the shaft a fan can be unfolded and attached to the middle of the shaft. The whole cane has to be moved to fan the air. American patent 1882.

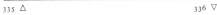

335 △   336 ▽

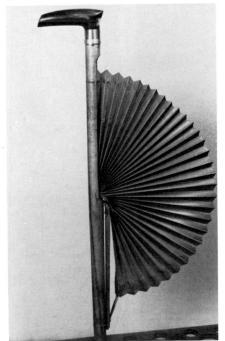

337   Long ivory handle (detail), heavily carved with
flowers and monogram. Long ivory ferrule on ebony
shaft. Well patinated. German or French, dated 1901.
Height 22 cm.

338   This ivory knob is decorated with roses, leaves
and rococo revival symbols. Probably an umbrella
handle converted into a lady's cane. Possibly from
Dieppe, France. End of 19th century.

339   Elongated ivory handle, ending in an oval knob,
which can be used as support. The garland of flowers
and leaves is carved from the full tusk. Provenance not
(as usually stated) Erbackh im Odenwald. Probably
middle 19th century.

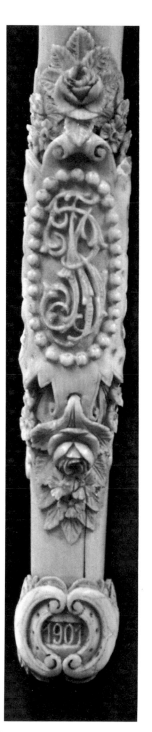
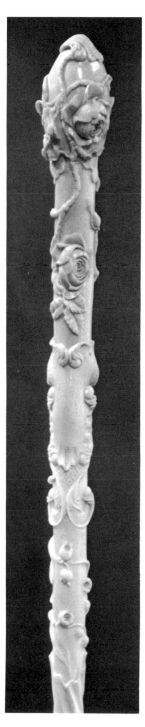
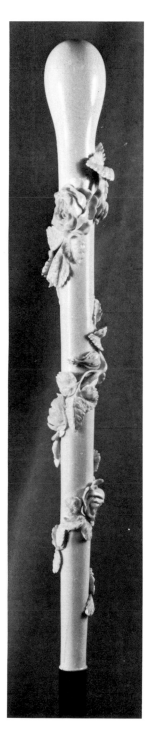

340, 341 *Lady's bust with hat and scarf in riding costume. ivory. Very decorative, appealing piece with strong expression. Beautiful patina. Probably German, prior to World War I. Height 13 cm.*

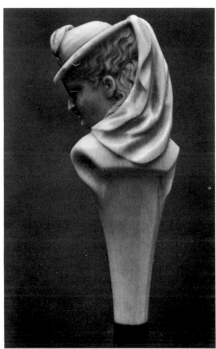

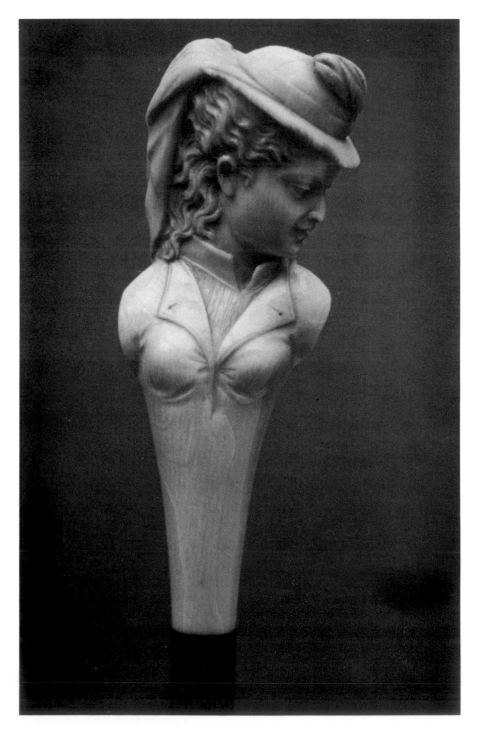

342-344 *Fully sculptured image of Lorelei, the rock, vines and an inscription "Loreley." Beautiful female nude with comb and harp, both upper arms decorated with bangles. Naturalistically executed at the end of the 19th century. height 13.5 cm.*

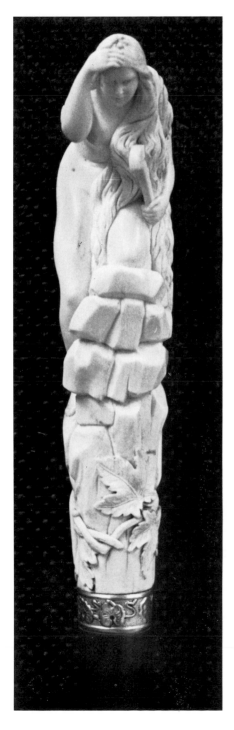
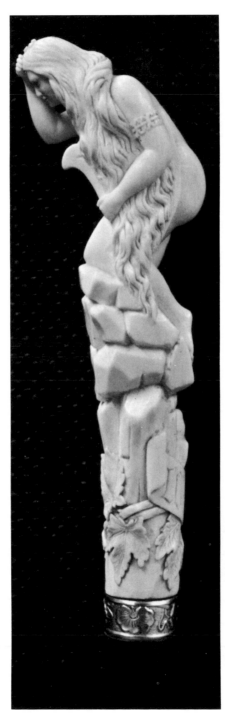
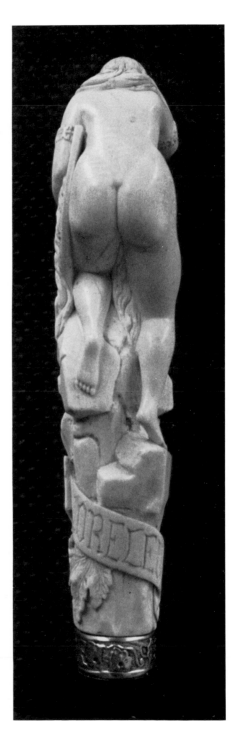

345 *Art Nouveau silver cane handle with female bust and head in the style of Alfonse Mucha. With rich, very detailed hair and floral ornaments. Both handles are full. Length of handle 11 cm.*

346 *Reclining nude, one hand covering her breast as if covering in shame, legs hidden in flower, which turns the ivory piece into a well fitting handle. Probably Dieppe, France, 18th century or early 19th century.*

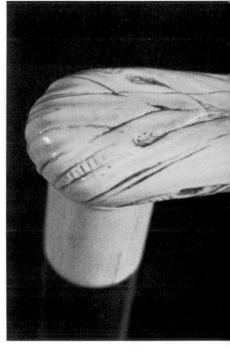

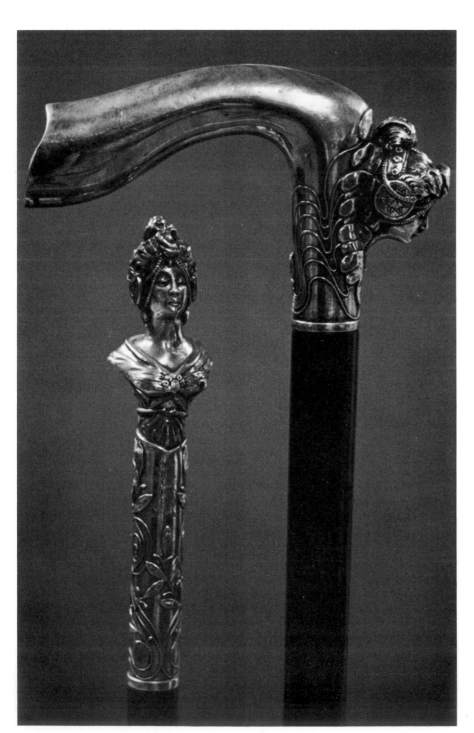

347   Naked nymph or similar mythological female fetching water from a spring. Very fine and expressive ivory piece. Wide ornamental silver band, knotted wood shaft.

348   Naked, backwards curving Eve or seductive female with snake. Expressive, well colored brown bronze. The female figure is a curved handle, fitting well in hand. Turn of the 20th century. Height 8 cm.

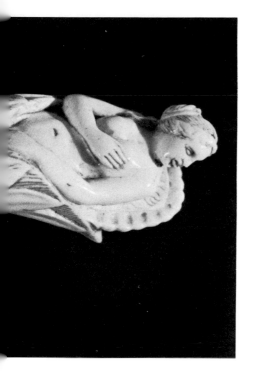

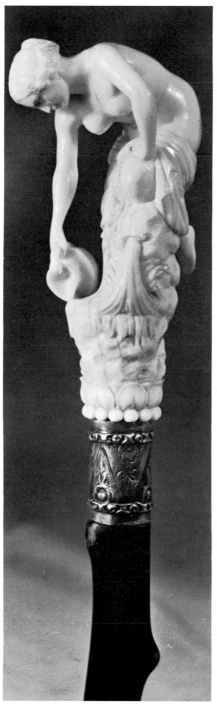

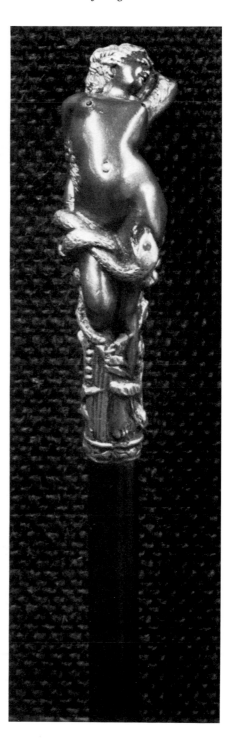

349 *Love in the chicken coop. Figures made of gilded bronze. Quite heavy cane. 19th century. Length 6 cm.*

350 *Penis emerging from a fantastic flower. Sterling silver, made by the contemporary New York artist Ivaan of Toronto cast in the lost wax method. Richly ornate and pierced piece in the Art Nouveau style. A good walking stick, shaft made of Madagascar Palisander wood. Height 10.5 cm.*

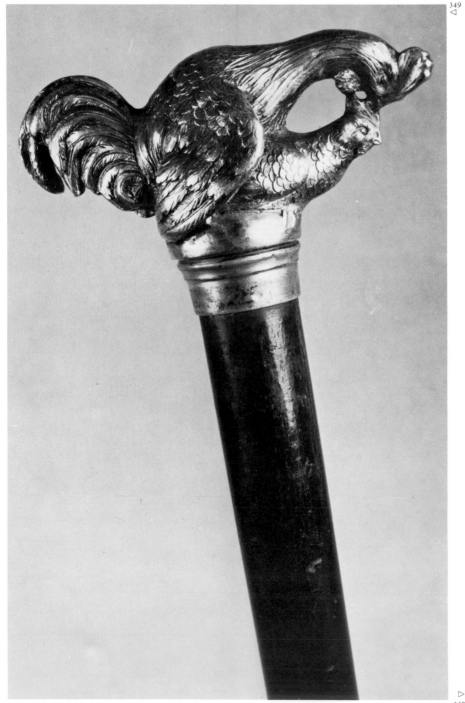

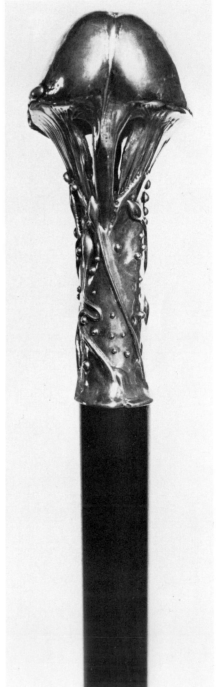

349 ◁

▷
350

351 Ball form knob, two bronze figures climb up the wooden shaft: Satan is pursuing a woman in nether garments. Frivolous work from the turn of the 20th century. Height of figure 8 cm.

352 The knob end in a turned wooden lid which can be removed: a miniature carving inside shows a love making scene. The image reminds one of the automaton movements of erotic pocket watches, which until 1815 were made in Switzerland and France. Diameter 4 cm.

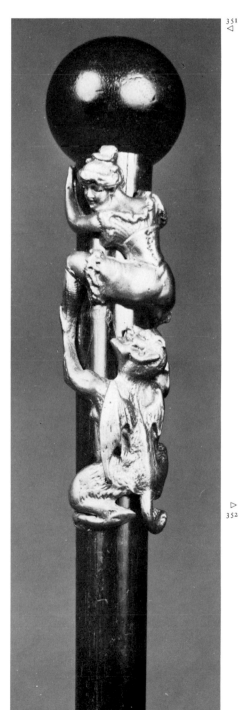

351

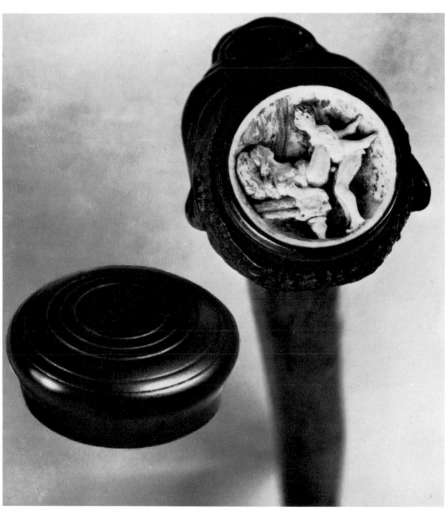

352

353-357 *For over 130 years this cane company in Allgau (Switzerland) was owned by the Egle family; however, after Johann Egle it will stop producing canes. In 1920 Johann Egle started his cane making apprenticeship and has been making canes ever since. Master Egle shows how, on the lathe, a square piece of wood turns into a cylinder and how the grater (illustration 354) removes all imperfections. Illustrations 355 - 357 show wooden handles, the inventory for hunting and souvenir sticks and the ever popular walking sticks, the illustrated ones are still missing their ferrules.*

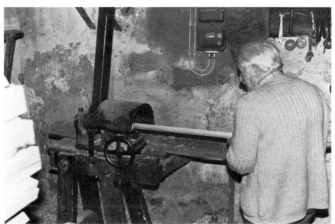

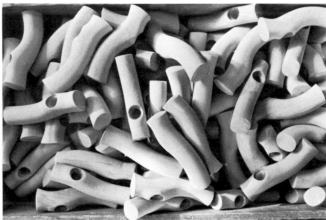

353 △   354 ▽   355 △

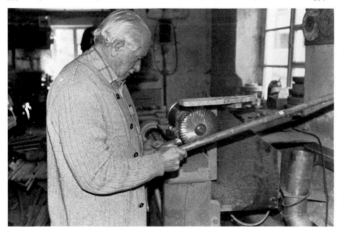

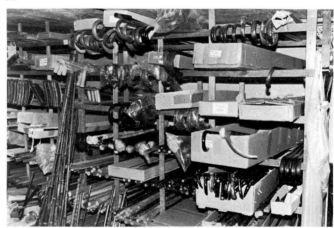

356 △   357 ▽

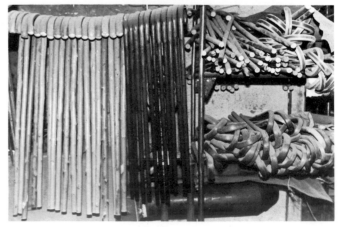

The Anatomy of the cane and its materials

Like every other object, a walking cane has its own terminology: particular terms for each of its components and part. As a practical guide for the study of auction catalogues and foreign language literature, the English terminology is expanded with corresponding terms in German and French.

Cane or walking stick	= Spazierstock	= canne
handle	= Griff	= pommeau or poignee
collar or ferrule	= Ring or Band	= bague or virole
shaft or shank	= Schuss	= jonc or fut
ferrule	= Zwinge oder Absatz	= ferrule

The handle

It is made of many different materials and in many different forms. We have already seen the knob, which is the oldest handle form. In its simplest form it is a plain metal lid, usually in metal, which covers the end of the shaft. In German and French terminology it is called Knauf or Knopf and pommeau or bouton.

Just as early, but disappearing as a model during the 19th century, is the Bec de Corbin. This French word for "raven's beak" is used internationally.

Curved handles are called crutches. The German term is Kruecke, which comes from the word Kringel, which means curve or bend. The English and German term originate in the same language family. There are several variations of the English crutch handle: the Opera style handle (German: Fritz kruecke) and the T-shaped handle with rounded ends (German: Derby kruecke). In French the crutch handle is pommeau en forme de tau or bequille.

If the handle is curved only in one direction, rounded or straight, this simple crutch is called cross hook (straight) or crook handle (curved). The German terminology is Haken (straight) or Rundhaken (curved). In France the cross hook is called Courbe, the crook handle is called Recourbe.

In old cane catalogues sometimes one can find the bell handle, which is in between the cross hook and crook handle.

The leg crook type with an elegant, narrow crook (= shepherds staff) was illustrated earlier as a paper cane (see illustration 53).

Another handle type is the thumb stick. The characteristic of this handle is its Epsilon shape. Similar canes are used by hunters to rest the gun or rifle. A well made crook handle should have the crook end higher than its base at the shaft; if handle and shaft are two pieces, the significant line is the collar. Carved handles are called figural or fantastic handles, or are called after the subject or the material used.

The collar

The ring covers the connection between handle and shaft on a two piece cane, or it is meant as a visual separation on a one piece cane. It also can give some strength to the handle. There is some terminological confusion in English: Ferrule, from the Latin viriola or the Scottish virl, also means iron ring, thus sometimes the ring is called a ferrule. With simple canes this ring is silver, aluminum, nickel, brass or copper. Better canes use artistically braided silver thread. These braid works were made by female workers in larger factories as piece-work, one of those factories specializing in the braided ring was R. Barthel in Berlin. Silver and gold rings can help us identify and date the cane based on the hallmarks. The rings made at the atelier of Carl Fabergé intrigue with their translucent enamel over engine turned metal. Rings made of ivory, antlers, rams horn, wood or leather are also known.

The ring should always be placed on the upper third of the cane, frequently it is the place for initials, inscriptions or the owner's armorial crest.

The shaft

The German term for the shaft of a cane is Schuss, and is probably derived from Schoessling, which is "a straight growing, young off shoot of a bush or tree" according to a large dictionary of the German language, which is missing the term "Schuss." Usually the shaft of a cane is made of wood. One distinguishes the natural shafts, which are off shoots either with or without the bark and the shafts made of core wood, where the tree trunk is cut into square timber prior to any other processing. Core wood shafts are always straight whereas the natural shafts have be straightened by bending.

Besides those, shafts can be made of many different materials, of which in illustrations 59 and 60 (pages 104 and 105) twenty different examples are shown: from paper to black coral, from sting ray to ox haunch.

The ferrule

The lower end of the cane is protected or decorated by an end piece, which is called Zwinge in German, deriving its name from Zwinge, Zusammendruecken, to press into something. Ferrules as protective pieces are usually made of metal, either wrought iron or brass. Due to muddy road conditions at the time, early canes have very long ferrules. Later ferrules are made of brass and iron, in a way, that the brass ring folds around the shaft and a little iron plate is soldered to the brass ring with a soft metal thread. This method has the advantage that a worn iron plate can be easily replaced in a way similar to the worn heel of a shoe. The form of the ferrule depends on the use of the cane: a walking and mountain cane has a pointed tip. If the ferrule of a strolling canes is made of horn or ivory, it is referred to as heel. This type of end piece has to be well attached to the shaft and have a conical shape to avoid the breaking and splintering of the cane and to look aesthetically appealing. The plastic ferrule is strikingly functional.

Small encyclopedia of cane woods

The majority of shafts is made of wood. Most of them are cut out of tree trunks, turned and polished slightly tapering toward the lower end. In earlier times many local woods were used. Natural wood canes from

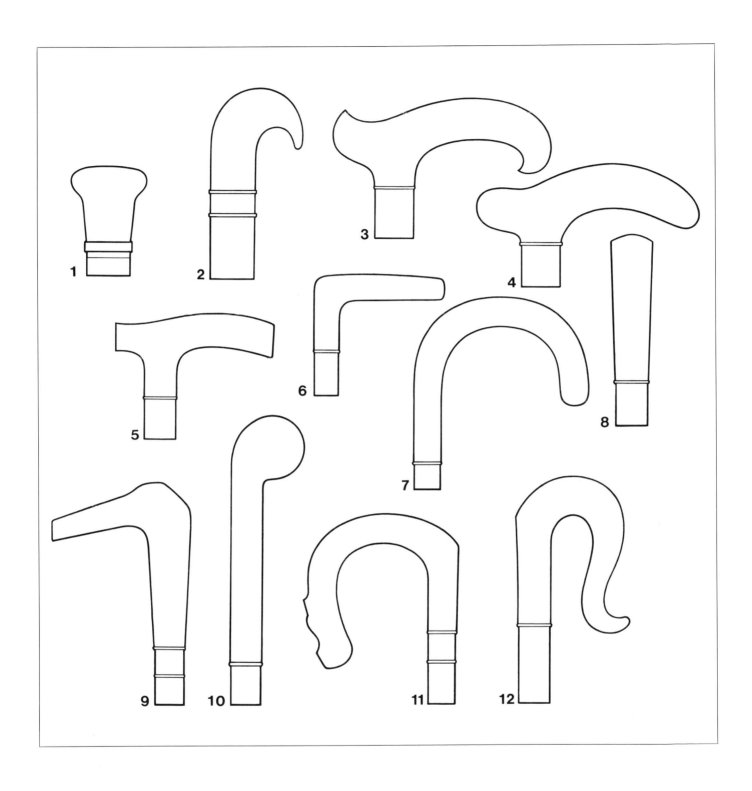

Fig. 52 Handle terminology and forms: 1 Knob; 2 Bec de Corbin; 3 Crutch Handle; 4 Rounded Crutch Handle or T-shaped Handle; 5 Opera Style Handle; 6 Cross Hook; 7 Crook Handle; 8 Straight Handle; 9 Hunting Hook; 10 Pistol Shaped Handle; 11 Shepherd's Staff - Neck Crook; 12 Shepherd's Staff - Leg Crook.

off shoots were used for unique folk art pieces, or as mass produced walking sticks.

Exotic canes usually use core wood, except for naturally grown canes. In industrial production the use of the woods has shifted: European woods are mainly used for handles, the exotic woods, which are easily machine treated, are mainly used for shafts.

1. European woods

Ash tree: Has a smooth grey bark, which is easily hurt, thus ash trees are either used without bark or cut from core wood.

Beech tree: The white beech tree is ideal for shafts, it is finely grained, light, tough and strong. Can be very nicely polished. The red beech tree is darker and porous and therefore less suitable but much cheaper.

Birch tree: The burl wood from Sweden and Finland has a very decorative graining, but is hard to work with and breaks easily. Bright yellowish color with flamed pattern. Almost exclusively used for handles.

Bruyere: The root wood of the arica arborea, also used for pipe heads, heavy, pale reddish brown and grained, for carved handles. Can not be bent.

Cherry wood: Earlier used for L shaped canes: the branch as handle, the off shoot as shaft. Later used as handle and shaft. The Viennese term is king wood. The color is almost white with reddish shine, well structured. Tough, strong wood with the highest specific weight of its class. Characteristic: dense, regular knots.

Chestnut tree: The majority of the walking sticks are made of off shoots of the chestnut tree. Either used smooth as grown in nature or scarred by cutting with a pair of tongs. Since the end of the 19th century this wood has the trade name "kongo." It is the least expensive wood.

Hazel tree: Always used with the smooth bark, with is greenish-yellow or silver grey. Not very strong wood. Better than the off shoots are young rooted trees.

Maple: Fascinates with its almost white color. Used mainly for handles, in earlier times whole canes.

Mistletoe: Raised in large cultures around Paris, mistletoes were pruned with special tongs during growth periods, resulting in either orderly or erratic growing shoots, which were the sensation at the World Fair in 1890. The skinned branches are silky shining and yellowish red, the wood is hard and fine and can be bent into a smooth crook.

Oak tree: The off shoot of a evergreen oak is an ideal shaft, the nicer the grooves and the fewer branches, the more expensive. The German oak does not have this advantage. Trunks of young oaks with the root as handle are rare.

Pear tree: Very dense and hard wood, reddish-brown with a touch of pink in color. Industrially produced canes use pear tree wood only for handles, in folk art some entire canes.

Sour Cherry tree: Relative of the cherry tree, the most famous natural cane with bark was cultivated in Lower Austria and Hungary. The handle is not cut from the root, but from the artificially thickened tip of the three year old tree. The bark is very thin, smooth and reddish brown, the wood is hard, dense and heavy. Cherry tree wood from Baden (a town in Lower Austria) smells like woodruff.

2. Exotic woods

These tropical woods are rare and nowadays are not allowed to be exported. Often they have trade or fantasy names which do not correspond to their botanical names and differ from country to country. They are frequently lacquered to hide imperfections in the wood.

Amaranth: Also known as purple ebony. Grows in northern Brazil and Guyana. The color is from reddish brown to purple, the splint wood (= the most recent year ring) is white and in strong contrast. Heavy, very fine porous wood, hard to work with.

Cocobolo: Characteristic with a dark fine pattern in the reddish-yellow wood. Grows in Costa Rica and Nicaragua, uneven growth.

Ebony woods: Black, real ebony is very strong and heavier than water. May come from Africa, Madagascar, Ceylon and India (= Bombay Ebony). The latter may be very inflexible. Grayish black is the Gabun or Camerun wood. More important for cane production is the brown, very decorative Makssar-ebony wood (Koromandel) from Celebes, either polished or stained black. Imitation ebony are black stained local woods, which can be identified by their lower weight.

Grenadill: The core wood is dark brown, almost black colored; therefore, also called black wood, very high specific weight, very hard, grows in Mozambique.

Iron woods: Collective term for various very hard woods, primarily from the Myrtazeen family (spice trees) like the nutmeg brown, very strong pigment wood, which can be bent into the finest natural wood cane. The flesh colored, very hard bull tree is also in this group.

Letter wood: The most expensive of the tropical woods. Very hard and heavy, sounds like metal and sinks like a stone in water. Brown reddish to pale pinkish color with spotted or wavering pattern (similar to snake skin, thus in German it is called "snake wood"). The English term is letter wood, because the pattern is similar to letters, the French term is amourette — favorite wood. Grows in Surinam and is used only for expensive handles, very rarely for a whole cane.

Palisander: Also called Jacaranda, very dark, with a purple shimmer, fine pored and hard. Different weights depending on its origin (Madagascar, East India or Brazil). The most decorative is the Rio Palisander.

Partridge: Coffee brown wood with grain, reminding one of partridge feathers (therefore its name). Hard and sturdy. Grows in Brazil and Venezuela. See also partridge cane.

Pockwood: Also called Guajakwood or Lignum Vitae. Very heavy, very hard and greasy. Weak, pleasant smell. Dark brown, rare as cane wood, usually used for bowling balls.

Rose wood: Also called Tulip wood. Red-white striped color, soft smell of roses. Strong and dense. Grows in Brazil (Bahia).

3. Canes and Bamboos

Different types of bamboo were often used for canes and shafts. They were named either after their origin, like Tonkin, their appearance, like Pearl Bamboo, or they received a trade name, like Pepper Cane.

Jambea: also called Jambis, a relative of the pepper cane.

Distinction: They leave knots that are not parallel, but alternating diagonally to each other. Very often used in England.

Malacca: Also called Spanish cane, the classic cane wood of the 18th and 19th century. Very valuable, if the distance between leaves is longer than the shaft and the lower end is less than 23 mm thick. The authenticity of the bark is important, which can be seen on the "spine" of the cane. Malacca is not round, but has a light ridge on one side. If the shaft is as long as the cane, we have an "authentic cane." If the shaft contains a leaf knot, which is planed, and only part of the cane still has the bark, then the shaft is referred to as "three quarter or half authentic." The bark is strong, like a glaze, from a light yellow to a dark brown in color, often in one color, but also seen as having darker spots on a lighter background. The more regular the pattern, the nicer the cane, the higher the ridge, the higher the quality and the more interesting the reflection of light. The cane is flexible. In botanical terms, the Malacca cane is the off shoot of the Rotang-Palm which is similar to a vine that climbs other trees.

Manila cane: Similar to Malacca, it is from the Calamus family, but much shorter. Cheap, light cane wood of light color with brown spots, which are burnished and intensified. Strong and inflexible. Is usually used for handles.

Paper cane: trade name for bamboo, yellow from China, dark with light specks from Japan. Hollow, inflexible cane, which is traded with its root, because it lends the handle its characteristic asparagus-like appearance.

Partridge cane: Named because of the brownish black partridge feather pattern. Comes from a small east Asian Palm tree. Inflexible, stiff and hard. There are no leaf knots on the smooth shoots, which are offered with the root. The surface, different form the Calamus family is always treated and polished.

Pearl Bamboo: Its chinese name is Whangee. It is massive, elastic, can be bent yet is very strong. The knots are very closely spaced (about 6 cm) and have scars like fine threads. Charlie Chaplin's cane was made from this wood. The natural bark glaze is dense and hard.

Sugar cane: Refers to the wood of the sugar palm tree (arenga sacharitera). Very flexible and sturdy, with bark hard as glaze. Yellowish white color, which ends in black at the end of the shaft.

Tonkin cane: The most known of all cane sticks, hollow and divided by horizontal walls. Yellowish color, light weight, strong and cheap.

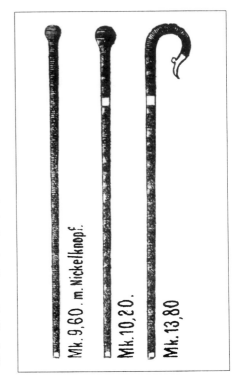

Illustration 53 Paper Cane from a catalogue from 1890. A favorite is the shepherd's crook. Prices are whole sale per dozen.

From mullein to paper cane

Many different botanical materials have been used for canes and handles. The feather weight Balsa wood has been covered with leather or snake skin or tropical nuts have been lined on a metal core. In Jersey, the 2 meter high stalks of a special cabbage are dried and converted into souvenir canes. The Viennese cane industry used the mullein, which can be higher than a human being in its third year, to make into a cane. The roots are knotty and form a natural handle, the pith filled stalk is very light.

An egg sized stone nut from Ecuador or Columbia is called vegetable ivory. Usually it is used for dice and buttons, but the very strong cream colored material has also been carved into handles.

The very "barky" rind of the cork-oak and the tea bush have inspired cane makers. The heavy marked shoots, rather thin in the tea bush, very thick in the cork-oak, are very sensitive to shock and are more useful for presentation than utility canes.

The tea rind is strong, but easily detaches from the wood, the cork rind is soft and gets bumpy. Canes made of pressed individual thin cork disks are useful. They are made in the same technique as paper canes. At first glance, they are very hard to identify, flexible, polished and in the colors of the paper canes. This can be either printed waste paper or high gloss paper, usually used for binding books. According to a patent from 1885 (DRP 30736), circular discs with a hole in the middle of each were cut from several layers of papers, strung on a flexible rod, condensed under high pressure, cut and sometimes lacquered. They are cheaper canes, but with a full handle they are useful weapons. Discharged soldiers frequently had a cane with a paper shaft ("Reservistenstoecke").

Ivory and other teeth

The term ivory is a general term for the teeth of elephant, mammoth, walrus, hippopotamus, sperm whale and pottwhale. From its linguistic root (Greek elephas and latin elephantus) and in colloquial terms, ivory comes from the African or Indian elephant. Carvers liked this material at all times, its translucency gives a special shine, and it was always used for handles. Elephant ivory as well as sperm whale tooth was made into shafts and seldom made into one piece canes. Due to endangered species laws and overreactions of legislative bodies, it is now hard to send antique ivory across borders.

Elephant ivory: The two heavy tusks of the elephant are slightly bent upwards and can reach a length of over 2 meters with a weight of up to 50 kilograms per tusk. The cross cut is either round or oval. Large tusks have a small hollow for the bone cone, on which the tusk sits, small tusks have a comparatively large hollow. The cross cut shows a net-like pattern, the length cut shows a line pattern. This pattern is unique to elephant tusks and it helps identify the material. The surface of the tusk is covered with a 5 mm thick bark, which is called cement. Ivory can be easily worked with, the hardness varies with its origin. The hard, so called glass bone comes from the African West coast, its reddish shimmer makes it a favored material for handles. Softer and easy to carve is ivory from East Africa. Because of its chalk-white color it is also referred to as light ivory. The shorter but thicker tusks of the Asian elephant have a finer patterned, harder and brighter ivory. It was exported to Europe only until 1900 — the best handles were made in Bautzen, Goerlitz and Dresden, in Nuernberg and especially Vienna. While England produced some nice handles, France's were insignificant. The earliest ivory imitations were made of cellulose or white artificial amber; nowadays, the imitations from plastic work frighteningly well. Optically they are only distinguishable by an expert. The safest identification, but not always possible, is with a gleaming needle.

Hippopotamus teeth: the lower corner teeth can be up to 60 cm long and weigh several kilos. The cement cover is too hard to work with and is removed with hydrochloric acid. The strong, bright white teeth will patinate well when used and turn into a characteristic brown. Further characteristics: If the nerve was carved, the cut looks like a seam. The teeth of the

African wart hog or the South East Asian wild boar were used as cheaper substitutes.

Mammoth ivory: very dry and chalky, usually from light to dark brown. Fossil ivory found in Siberia can be carved into a unique handle.

Walrus tusks: The downwards curved teeth of the walrus can be up to 1 meter long and weigh 6 kilograms per tusk. They are slightly curved, have grooves and are massive. The inflexible and glassy tusks are very hard and towards the core have inclusions which appear crystal-like. Their use for handles is much rarer than for elephant tusks.

Sperm whale teeth: The lower teeth of the always heavily hunted sperm whale are approximately 15 cm long and 5 cm thick and look similar to the end piece of a cucumber. Their use as handle material is almost always in combination with whale bone. Otherwise used for scrimshaw. (see illustration 70). The yellowish-white teeth develop a nice patina.

Narwhal tooth: The left tusk of the male whale can grow up to 2 meters, with a diameter of 10 cm on the thickest point. The right tusk is rarely developed, females do not have tusks. Different from any other teeth, the narwhal tooth is turned from bottom to tip, the grooves, when seen from the base always run from right to left. These grooves are the easiest way to differentiate a polished sperm whale tooth from elephant ivory: on the cream colored cane one can still see the grooves faintly running from right to left. The stick made from such a tooth is hollow except for a little section on the peak; the cave is filled by a nerve, which is a porous mass with a dark rim. The color of the tooth ranges form cream colored to brownish grey, untreated it has a rough surface. Inside it is ivory colored, patinated towards a cream color. For many centuries the narwhal was the most valued whale earth had to offer. It was the horn of the fairy unicorn, full of power, magic and strength. In 1612 it was one thousand nine hundred times more expensive than elephant ivory. Small wonder that it was used exclusively for scepter and presentation chalices (which rendered any poison harmless). There are also a few bishop's staffs made of narwhal tooth: the oldest one is in the Treasury in Vienna and belonged to Saint Rupert, the founder of Salzburg. The bishop's and abbot's staff in the Treasury of Saint Peter's in Salzbug (Austria) are from the 17th century. At this time the narwhal bias started, when it was realized that the material did not come from unicorns, but rather was the tooth of a sea animal. However, it never became competition for ivory: the tooth of the narwhal was always more special and exclusive. The first canes for noble men were made from narwhal. The Rosenborg castle in Kopenhagen owns the oldest narwhal cane, which had been given by Duke William of Weimar-Saxon to Frederick III of Denmark, a collector of unicorns and canes in 1641. Additional narwhal canes are in the Duke Anton Ulrich museum in Braunschweig (three examples) and in the Historical Museum of the Town of Frankfurt. All of them were made from the tip of the tooth, some keeping their natural form, other were turned to achieve a regular spiral marking. Guido Schoenberger has dated the treated canes as 18th century, the untreated ones either earlier or later. — Knobs, handles and ferrules are almost always made from another material: ivory, silver, tortoise or turned wood. One narwhal cane in my collection is made from one single piece: the knob, thicker than the shaft, is carved in the form of a closed flower bud, the opening for the nerve is closed with carved tooth material. Canes from narwhals are exclusive, rare and expensive, therefore there are many imitations made of plastic. These imitations, however, are lacking the nerve cave.

Whalebone: The largest animals on earth are the blue whales. Since they feed on tiny animals called krill, they need a device to filter their prey out of the water. For this they have baleen plates with fringes, which hang from the palate. Whale bone is the technical terms for treated baleen plates, which because of their elasticity, the way they can be bent and their strength, were an important material before plastic was invented. Canes were covered with polished or textured fish bone, the most valued whale bone was from the Nordic Right Whale (Balena mysticetus). A substitute for whale bone canes were Manila cane combined with a mixture of black paint, rubber and gutta percha mixed under pressure and heat. The trade name of this material was Wollosin. Successors of the fish bone cane were the ones made of Ebonite, a hard rubber with gutta percha mixture.

Whalebone and other bones

In America the term whale bone is used for the skeleton bones of whales and for baleen. The bones of whales were made into canes by the whalers. We can recognize canes made from jaw and ribs of the sperm or right whale by their porous dotted surfaces. They do not have the polished surface of ivory, but rather are bones with fine pores. The technique itself is called scrimshaw, from the old term scrimshanker, which meant "useless idler,": the items made of whale bones and teeth were considered useless, even if artistic. These carvings were so common that one could call them the universal occupation of a whaling ship's crew. By the way, fresh whale bone was so soft that it could easily be grated and carved. The spines were used for canes, by stringing the vertebra on steel poles.

Handles and assembled shafts were made from the front and back foot bones of cows, the most expensive ones came from South America. They also can be distinguished from ivory by the pores. Horse bones have a dense but thin wall, the inside being very porous. Deer bones are hard and inflexible with small cells, useful only for small handles. The yellowish color of bone can be bleached to a bright white.

Horns and antlers

Horns are the headpiece and weapons of a group of animals, which are made of a thick, ever growing and hardening layer of skin. In the cane industry horn is used for handles, ferrules and sometimes for shafts, since the material can be softened by heating, bent and molded by pressure, turned and carved.

The most frequently used horn is buffalo horn. Buffalo horns are divided into: 1. Caphorn, milky white to light grey, the lighter, the more valuable. 2. Brazil horn, black. 3. Siam horn, silver grey with green shimmer, which makes it very desirable, and very large — all horns have a dark core stripe, in which the nerve is housed. The less the stripe is visible, the more valuable the cane.

Sheep's horn (trade name Belier) used for shepherd's staffs. Rams horn can be very easily molded and has a low tendency to splinter or rip. Chamois horn was used in its natural form for walking sicks, sometimes also antelope horns. The long and pointed horn of the African pike buck was sometimes made into a whole cane.

The rhinoceros horn does not have a bone base, but rather is solely a skin object, built from melted hairlike fibers. This will always distinguish it. The core, which is blackish in color, is very dense at the center. The colors range from green to pale blond, the nicer the pattern, the more expensive the horn. Canes entirely made of rhinoceros exist; because of the precious material, they are usually combined with gold. Rhinoceros horn can be very nicely carved (the Chinese are masters in that art), figural handles also exist. In Asia rhinoceros horn is considered an aphrodisiac, in Jemen stable handles must be made of rhinoceros horn. Rhinoceros horns are usually 50 cm long (exemptions up to 1 meter) and are valued in German Marks at 20,000 per kilogram on the Singapore market.

Hartshorn is the trade name for the antlers of elk, deer, moose and reindeer. Antlers are not horn, but a bone-like, massive substance, which may be carved but not worked with or bent. Only for handles, usually including the first ending. (?) At the base of the antler a disk like ring with pearled rim forms which is called a rose. For hunting canes the rose is usually carved with crests and reliefs. During the Biedermeier period hartshorn was used for nose men (Illustrations 114-116).

Tortoise is real horn: the upper plate of the torso of water turtles from Asian waters. The material is denser and more bendable than any other horn. The spotted pattern and its translucency make it a material for luxury articles. Since it can be softened with heat and welded together, it can be turned into handles and whole canes. Besides amber, tortoise was the most cherished turner's product. Real tortoise handles and canes are welded, an inner sheep's horn core (= Belier) is plated with tortoise. It is applied under pressure. Bond tortoise is the most sought after.

The main places for tortoise production were Paris in France, Vienna in Austria, Naples in Italy and Ober and Niederramstadt in Hesen and Nurnberg for Germany.

The best horn canes were also made in Paris; the best compound canes were from Tuscany. The multi-colored horn discs, referred to in English as washers, were made from cut horn.

Mother of pearl is made of the inner layer of the shell of oysters and abalone. The polished flattened plane has a nice reflecting color, because the light passes to various layers, is broken into rainbow

From Mother of Pearl to Ox pizzle

colors and is reflected. Canes are inlaid with mother of pearl, the Japanese artists dynasty Shibayama have used mother of pearl combined with coral since the late 18th century, with lacquer and gold as inlay on ivory handles.

Coral and amber are very rare as handles. A few lady's umbrella and cane handles do exist as long and straight canes which are carved with floral motifs. Amber was used in the 18th century by the Amber Master Goehlert in Berlin, who advertised cane knobs. The Prussian Cane knob producer Biet, who also worked for the court, combined amber with coconut shell and mother of pearl.

Hippopotamus skin was made into canes in Zansibar. Quoting from a trade revue of 1885 "The most beautiful riding whips and walking canes can be cut out of one hippopotamus skin in hundreds, the diameter is over 2.5 cm, and the articles cut from one can be polished nicely, which makes them translucent and yellow brown in color."

Rhinoceros skin was imported by German, Belgian and French makers and also made into canes: thin iron cores were either braided with leather or the leather was warmed, stretched and pressed on the glue covered iron stick.

Ox pizzle is the name for canes made from the dried penis of a bull or from dried and braided ligaments, usually around a metal core. The German term Ziemer comes from the word Sehne, as a synonym for penis. At the end of the 19th century the two ox pizzle manufacturers were Emil Weiss in Berlin and J.G. Dennstedt in Muhlhausen/Thuringen.

Porcelain handles

The 18th century porcelain companies also made stock handles, which were very popular. The hero poem "Rennomist" written in 1744 by Zacharias has the following verses:

"His cane from India is adorned by a special handle
a Lady's head in porcelain from Meissen;
the dead ceramic gave pleasure to the eye
charm is on the forehead, malice in the eye."

Walter Stengel writes in "Guckkasten Altberlin," that "Lady's faces" were very popular handle forms. "An example from the Wegelschen factory, in whose auction catalogue from November 25, 1765 canes knobs and handles with or without faces are listed, with a purple scarf and a white cap, covered by a black scarf, which adds up to the not idealized but rather realistic portrait of a good Berlin middle class woman. The later styles of royal manufacture, which had to cater to a different group, do not have this closeness to life. The realism was unimportant, with the exception of a model which was 'like branches,' an unusual subject for the material. In the lost/found archives of Hannover a porcelain handle covered with gilded flowers on a lacquered thorn shaft was listed on January 14, 1766. The porcelain knob disappears after the rococo."

Contradictory information is given by the VEB Porcelain Manufacture in Meissen: "cane handles were part of the production line until the '30s of this century, which also means that no separate archival entries about designers and painters were kept. The molds are still stored, but have not been used since then." The models are X75 (circa 1844) handle with face and veil; model G133 (circa 1865) dog's head as knob; K 191 (circa 1876) plain knob; L 168 and L187 (circa 1877-1880) crooked handle and handle with pug's head. Without date M109 plain small knob and B199 plain handle.

It is difficult to date and research porcelain cane handles. They never had porcelain marks and always were copied without any concern about copyrights. According to Max von Boehm the Porcelain Company of King Karl III offered 18 different Cane knobs from 1 to 60 Ducat a piece. The lady with the mask is offered as a needle box by Chelsea, why not also as a cane knob? It was certainly offered in Vienna, and St. Cloud had it in its program line. The company in Nymphenburg offers today Bustelli No. 528 young girl's bust, No. 587 Male head, No. 816 harlequin and No. 2077 girl's head. H. Hofmann says in his book about the company "the form inventory of 1760 lists '6 types of Knobs;' the price list from 1767 lists under accessories a 'cane knob with female face' and a 'knob with Jewish head' (which is a Bustelli's male head). They also included pieces 'knob with male face in the style of a goose beak,' 'knob as crocodile' and 'knob pet d'corbine' could not be confirmed. The 'goose beak' is a goose sitting on the head biting the nose. The no longer existent (also not in illustrations) 'pet d'Corbine' probably had the handle form 'bec de Corbin.'" (see fig. 52)

The Federal Company of Berlin made some knobs during the 18th century, among them the "female face" with or without veil or mask. Erich Koellmann writes in his book about Berlin Porcelain: "The decision, whether the listed pieces 'Amazones,' 'Shaft-Knob' or other knobs, which are painted with flowers, fruit, 'ovidic,' 'Vatau,' 'purple children,' 'with green or blue figure and landscapes' or similar treated sword and knife handles, are actually Berlin products will be difficult, because marks are always lacking and the small size of the items makes an in-depth knowledge of appearance of material and glaze, ornamental characteristics and colors and brush strokes difficult."

Sevre, according to its archival curator, never made cane knobs; there are none at the Museum in Limoge and ones from Delft are unknown to the author.

Silver handles were made in four different techniques: 1. silver sheets were pressed on forms (= negative forms) and the 2 pieces were soldered together. They are hollow inside and were filled with stone cement. These kind of handles were, depending on the thickness of the sheet, made of 30 to 100 grams of silver. — 2. They are full cast in a form. These knobs weigh approximately 200 grams. Com-

Silver and other metals

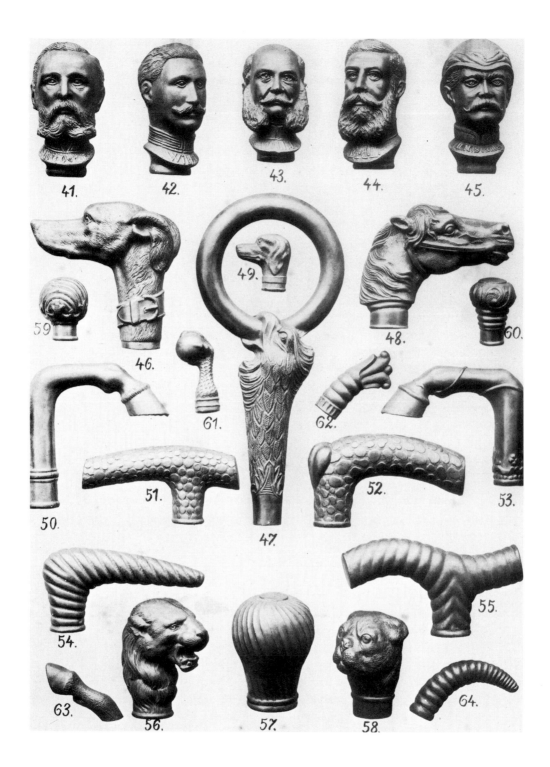

Fig. 54 *Catalog page from the Metal Foundary of Rich. Heinig & Company, Glauchau in Saxony, dating from 1900. The catalog featured a variety of handle forms including knobs and figurals.*

panies which specialized in these knobs and similar silver articles were in Pforzheim (e.g. Emil Scheidel) and in Gmuend/Schwaben (e.g. B. Ott and Joseph Pauser). — 3. The lost cast form is made with a wax model, which is destroyed during the procedure, thus each piece is unique. — 4. The metal is chased. Precious metals such as gold and silver expand and the metal is chased on a soft undersurface (such as pitch) with a hammer and chisel into lines, pattern, and ornamental and figural reliefs. Eighteenth century gold buttons were crafted in such a way. The most expensive pieces employed tri-color gold. Some types of silver handles were gold plated or made of new silver (a copper-zinc-mangan alloy) or Alpaca (copper-zinc-nickel alloy). The Richard Heing Company in Galauch offered in its catalogue of 1900 259 differed handles made of Britannia metal. (see Fig. 54)

In the 20th century, seamless metal canes with wood grain pattern were made in the most realistic way. In light colors for lady's at sea resorts, they could be unscrewed to fit in travelling suitcases and last but not least as advertisements, which the metal industry gave as New Year's gifts. The main manufacturer was the Kronprince AG in Ohligs. The Jacob Haish Wire Company gave braided wire mesh canes as gifts during the World's Fair in St. Louis. According to the wire mesh expert Jack Glover, Sunset, Texas, nine example of those are known to exist in collections.

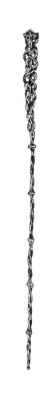

Fig. 55 Barbed wire cane, an example of the form from Jack County/Texas, dated 1975.

Artificial materials in the cane industry

It is plastic products which can replace precious materials such as ivory, tortoise, horn or amber. They do not have to be perfect imitations. The company H.C. Meyer Jr. in Hamburg-Harburg purchased the hard rubber patent from Charles Goodyear, because they heard that it would push whalebone from the market. Canes and handles were made form the new material; in a period catalogue they were offered as "real Indian rubber". The material was further improved, became even more similar to horn and was called ebonit. Ebonit handles could be worked with similar techniques as horn handles.

The synthetic material celluloid was mainly used for umbrella handles and, because it was flammable, it soon was replaces by cellon. It can be formed, modeled and pressure welded. Galalith (= artificial horn) was introduced to Germany in 1897 as D.R.P. No. 32293 and was produced by Hoff & Co. in Harburg/Elbe "the oldest and most competent artificial horn manufacturer on earth." "It has the same qualities and therefore can be used as the most precious natural products ivory and tortoise." Galalith canes were produced in any color. One can make either canes or handles, which was done more often.

Synthetic resin was invented in 1907 and turned into "the ideal product for cane and umbrella handles." Unbreakable, it could imitate ivory, tortoise and horn in "extraordinary ways." The trade names were Ambrasit, herolith, leukorit or vigorit.

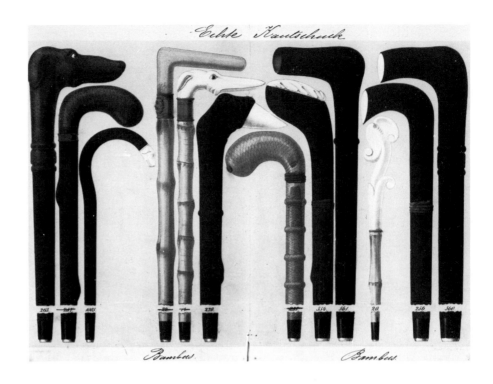

Fig. 56 Catalog pages from the firm H.C. Meyer, advertising a variety of canes in hard rubber = Genuine India-Rubber, 1852.

Glass canes

Transparent, with colorful bands either interlaced or overlaid, and often turned or filled with colorful love pearls, glass canes were more like class emblems or luck charms in cane form. They have either knobs, crooks or leg crooks and in that respect are perfect models of walking canes: glass blowers used them to show off their skills, similar to the air bubble filled glass balls, which later developed into paperweights. George Soanes tells in his "curiosities of literature" in 1847 about the glass makers in Nailsea, Somerset, that they had glass sticks displayed in their apartments, which were dusted every day and which shielded against diseases, especially fever.

In Belgium, young men took "glass luck charms" to their military recruitment, according to Dieter W. Banzhaf. Through a small hole they had been filled with alcohol. If the young man was recruited, he would knock off the end and drink the alcohol. Daniel Spoerri tells about an old custom in France: soldiers, when went into war, would take the cut off piece of a glass cane, which they had left behind, as a talisman. Illustration 69 shows a collection of recruit canes form Normandy.

During guild processions the glass makers of Bristol and Newcastle took glass canes as signs of their guild. Glass canes were made since the middle of the 18th century.

When the cane industry had invented their most useful machines, when canes could be easily bent, turned and fashioned by machine, when woods could be colored in depth and they were impregnated for better durability, the cane industry came to its end. In 1929 265 cane manufacturers existed and over 100 companies specializing in handles. Their production included mountain canes, patent canes, strolling canes and lady's and children canes (almost all of companies offered them). The companies were concentrated in three areas: Lindewerra on the Werra had 17, Buergel in Thueringen had 14 and Eschwegen in Hessen had 11 companies. Earlier canes were made all over Germany, with the exception of Pommern and Mecklenburg.

The following specialized trades were included under the general term "Cane and umbrella maker:" mounter, frame maker, round turner, umbrella worker, umbrella repairer, parasol maker, shaft maker, shaft bender, whip maker, turner, umbrella maker, cane whip maker, round bender, inlay maker, cane stainer, cane rasper, cane turner, cane maker!

Did one ever see a soccer player on his way to the stadium with a cane? No, and because he's used to it now, he does not carry a cane at any other occasion. And now the modern means of transportation: bicycle and motorcycle, or car! When they are used it is impossible to carry a cane. The following count was made on a holiday on a main road into town: within 15 minutes 386 cars, usually for 4 people. 11 buses with 30 to 60 people, 422 motorcycles and 303 bicycles; approximately 2000 men without cane. And at another occasion: of 100 men who entered a public park, only 9 were carrying a cane, 47 had a camera in hand and were therefore without cane, the remainder without reason. Many these men were carrying brief cases, which according to Max von Boehm, are the main reason for the canes demise: ever since every better gentlemen feels obliged to carry a briefcase, even if it contains nothing but the newspaper and a snack, the cane was pushed aside, probably because most men are incapable of carrying two pieces at the same time without inconveniencing themselves and others.

A bad economic situation, changing social and traffic situations, a new trend and finally the Third Reich, during which the strolling cane was a symbol for the "old system," have made the cane disappear within a few years. The following war and the shortage of basic materials killed a whole trade: the occupations cane maker, bender and turner do not exist any more. A few companies continue to produce walking sticks, crutches and canes for the blind. Trendy canes will not be available in the near future, because the true know-how will die; despite the fact that new canes come from Italy, some with watches or included telescope; despite the fact that one can still order a cane in England. These are oddities such as trendy custom-made shoes, cautious experiments in reviving the past. Will they be successful?

To guard the past, this has been successfully done by collectors.

The end of the age of the cane to its revival by collectors

The cane as collector's item

Canes always have been collector's items, a phrase, which is written fast, but hard to prove. Were Voltaire, who owned 80 canes, or Count Bruehl, who owned 300, cane collectors or men of their time who were eccentric in matters of trend? Can one nowadays call a man who owns and wears 150 ties a tie collector?

Different from old nativities, textiles or carnival masks, to name but three areas — not a single cane collection can be mentioned, which could be visited. The German Museum guide does not include the category cane. Even if researching, one only gets vague information: Dali has collected canes, the cane collection of Sir Winston Churchill can be seen in Chartwell; the Smithsonian Institution in Washington DC has many canes; the collection of Jay de Rothschild has been sold at Sotheby's Monaco. And canes in museum collections have to be looked for to be found.

As a careful observer of the international antiques and collector's market, one could notice that over the past ten years more and more women and men in Germany, Switzerland, Austria, Italy and the Near East have started to collect canes. France and England always had a cane tradition, and in the United States the cane collector's virus has only started in the last 2 to 3 years. The entry is usually the same: grandfather's old canes are unearthed, considered very decorative and additional ones are bought. Whoever wanted a larger selection had to travel to London or Paris, where there are specialized stores. In Paris and Chartres specialized cane auctions are held, at Sotheby's and Christie's, where they offer more and more in objects de vertu sales. Nowadays one can also find canes in this country. No fair or antique market is complete without a stand full of canes, which usually come from England, but more and more canes with German or Austo-Hungarian provenance are offered. The higher demand has also increased the offering: a phenomenon which is also known from other collecting areas. Very nice objects come to the market, but at a price.

The most expensive are canes which overlap with other collecting areas. The carved canes of the Zulu's or Maori's are sought by tribal art collector's and seem unreachable for the cane collector. A watch cane can catch a watch collector's attention, who is willing to pay a high price. A camera cane lures the photography collector, and some system canes (violin canes) are so rare that they have a very high price. Canes with gold handles have a high material value and almost a magnetic attraction. Despite the acceleration of the cane market, imitations are rare. Imitation materials do exist: gold, which turns out to be a different material, or imitation ivory, but this can be confirmed when looking at the cane or it can be returned, if it has been purchased from a reputable dealer. Flea markets can be dangerous, if one is unexperienced, and it is not advisable to purchase from catalogues at auction without inspection. A number of ivory copies do exist, which are made into handles, but are offered as imitation. Sometimes, they can change into real antique pieces.

One frequently can find self-made pieces: just as in pre-cane collecting times, cane knobs were made into seals, now the opposite is made and seals are made into cane knobs. This is not that tragic: if the objects originally had been made by artists, very often the same artist would have also made cane knobs. The carved knife handles from the 18th century can not be distinguished from a cane handle from the same period.

The collectors can not agree on whether to add a missing shaft. Of course a beautiful handle with a period malacca shaft is the collector's dream. A one piece cane can not be added to. But if the wooden shaft of a cane is damaged, is scratched or painted over, this will influence the appearance of the cane. It should be either surface treated or replaced, just as the original owner of the cane would have done. It is similar to collecting "old timers:" the rust is removed and dirt is not considered patina. It means that one takes care of one's collection and does not let it collect dust. Dust can settle in fine grooves and be very aggressive. Wooden canes can be impregnated, silver and rings should be polished every two months.

The presentation of canes is simple. In the beginning use a cane stand like the ones used in wardrobes. Later the canes have to be divided. More than 50 canes in one place do damage to the individual objects. I made this mistake and, in the meantime, have built a three row giant stand into a side room. It is my depot, from which I supply my changing exhibitions. The most beautiful pieces I always have around me. An interesting way to display simple canes is on a billiard stick holder.

Another problem are visitors: many people have the urge to touch everything but do not know how to handle canes properly. This can pose some danger for delicate and precious objects. But this problem has to be solved individually.

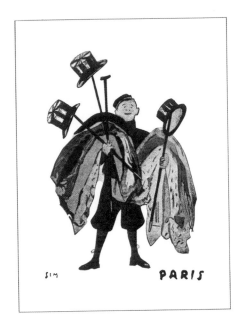

Fig. 57 Drawing of a turn of the twentieth century Paris cloak-room boy, signed SEM.

Bibliography

ALFA Catalogue: Arms of the World 1911. The Fabulous ALFA Catalogue of Arms and the Outdoors. Ed. by Joseph J. Schroeder, Jr. Chicago, Follett Publ. Northfield/Ill., Digest Books, 1972.

Amira, Karl von: Der Stab in der germanischen Rechtssymbolik. 1908.

Banzhaf, Dieter W.: Die gläsernen Glücksbringer. Englische und belgische Spazierstöcke aus einem ungewöhnlichen Material. In: Kunst & Antiquitäten, H. II, März/April 1981.

Banzhaf, Dieter W.: Schwäche für das 3. Bein. In: Expertise. Ärztezeitschrift für Sammeln, Kunst u. Kultur, 2/1980, S. 23–25.

Barton-Wright, E. W.: Self-Defence with a Walking-Stick. In: Pearson's Magazine, Vol. XI, Jan.–Juni 1901. Pub. Ed. Offices C. Arthur Pearson LTD. Pearson's Magazine Office, London.

Benker, Gertrud: Altes bäuerliches Holzgerät. München, Callwey Verlag, 1976. 207 S., Abb., Taf.

Bericht: Amtlicher Bericht über die Industrie-Ausstellung aller Völker zu London im Jahre 1851, v. d. Berichterstattungs-Kommission der Deutschen Zollvereins-Regierungen. 3. u. letzter Theil. § 142 Stöcke. Berlin, Mm. d. Innern, 1853.

Boehn, Max von: Das Beiwerk der Mode. München, Bruckmann Verlag, 1928. 277 S., 293 Abb., 16 Farbtaf.

Boothroyd, A. E.: Fascinating Walking Sticks. Foreword by Sir Gerald Nabarro. London/New York, White Lion Publ., 1973. 205 S., Abb.

Bradley Martin, Esmond u. Chryssee: Run Rhino Run. Intr.: Elspeth Huxley. Photogr.: Mohamed Amin. London, Chatto & Windus, 1982. 136 S.

Browning, Gertrude: The Cane as Art and Artifact. In: The Antiques Journal, Febr. 1973, S. 20–22, 52.

Buxa, Werner: Der Kampf am Wolchow und um Leningrad 1941–1944. Eine Dokumentation in Bildern. Dorheim, Podzun Verlag, 1969. 175 S.

Charlemont, J.: L'art de la boxe française et de la canne. Nouveau traité théorique et pratique. Paris, l'Académie de Boxe, 1899.

Dike, Catherine: Les Cannes à Système. Un monde fabuleux et méconnu. Paris, Ed. de l'Amateur, 1982. XII, 340 S., Abb.

Dite, Tibor: Stockflinten und Stockbüchsen. In: Deutsches Waffenjournal Nr. 12, Dez. 1975, S. 1382–1386.

Eelking, Baron von: Das Bildnis des eleganten Mannes. Ein Zylinderbrevier v. Werther bis Kennedy. Berlin-Grunewald, Herbig Verlagsbuchhdlg. »Walter Kahnert«, 1962. 254 S., Abb.

Exner, Wilhelm Franz: Das Biegen des Holzes, ein für Möbelfabrikanten, Wagen- und Schiffsbauer, Böttcher etc. wichtiges Verfahren. Mit bes. Rücksichtnahme auf die Thonetsche Industrie. 3., neubearb. u. erw. Aufl. v. Georg Lauboeck. Weimar, Voigt, 1893.

Fairholt, F. W.: Costume in England. A history of dress. London, Chapman and Hall, 1860. 607 S., Abb.

Fél, Edit u. Tamás Hofer: Husaren, Hirten, Heilige. Menschendarstellungen in der ungarischen Volkskunst. Corvinia Verlag, 1966. VIII, 69 S., 40 Taf.

Finkenstaedt, Helene u. Thomas: Stanglsitzerheilige und Große Kerzen. Stäbe, Kerzen und Stangen der Bruderschaften u. Zünfte in Bayern. Weißenhorn, Anton H. Konrad Verlag, 1968. 244 S., 80 Taf.

Flayderman, E. Norman: Scrimshaw and Scrimshanders. Whales and Whalemen. Ed.

by R. L. Wilson. New Milford/Conn. Flayderman, 1972. XII, 293 S., Abb.

Francesco, Grete de: Das Kleid des Arztes in drei Jahrhunderten (16., 17. u. 18. Jh.). In: Ciba Zeitschrift Nr. 11, Juli 1934, S. 363–369.

Fritzsch, Karl Ewald u. Friedrich Sieber: Bergmännische Trachten des 18. Jahrhunderts im Erzgebirge und im Mansfeldischen. Berlin, Akademie Verlag, 1957. V, 79 S., 31 Bildtaf. = Dt. Akademie der Wissenschaften zu Berlin. Veröffentlichungen des Instituts für dt. Volkskunde, Bd. 12.

Frost, Gordon Il.: Blades and Barrels: Six Centuries of Combination Weapons. El Paso/Texas, Walloon Pr., 1972.

Gentleman: Der Gentleman. Ein Herrenbrevier. Hrsg. v. F. W. Koebner. Unveränd., v. Hrsg. autorisierter Faksimiledruck der 1913 in Berlin ersch. Ausg. München, Rogner & Bernhard, 1976. 130 S.

Gong, Xia: Walking Sticks – Useful, Ornamental and Legendary. In: China Reconstructs, Aug. 1983, S. 64f.

Grant, David u. Edward Hart: Shepherds' Crooks and Walking Sticks. 2nd ed. Clapham, Dalesman, 1978. 48 S., Abb.

Happel, Jacob: Das Geräthfechten. Das Stock-, Stab-, Säbel- und Schwertfechten. Antwerpen, Brünners Druckerei, 1877. IX, 100 S., 51 Abb.

Hardwick, Paula: Discovering Horn. Guildford/Surrey, Lutterworth Pr., 1981. 192 S., Abb.

Hassan, Ali: Stöcke und Stäbe im Pharaonischen Ägypten. München, Deutscher Kunstverlag, 1976. Münchner Ägyptologische Studien, Heft 33.

Heimisch, Carl: Handwerksbrauch der alten Steinhauer, Maurer und Zimmerleute, Stuttgart, Verlag Konrad Wittwer, 1872.

Holliday, Robert C.: Walking-Stick Papers. New York, 1918.

Howard, Merriden: Walking stick wonderland. In: Pearson's Magazine, Juli–Dez. 1897. Pub. C. Arthur Pearson LTD. »Pearson's Magazine Office«, Henrietta St, W. C.

Journal des Luxus und der Moden. Hrsg. v. F. J. Bertuch u. G. M. Kraus. Bd. 1 1786 – Bd. 17 1802.

Katalog: Couleurstudenten in der Schweiz. Schweizerisches Museum für Volkskunde Basel. Ausstellung 1979/80. Führer durch das Museum für Völkerkunde u. Schweizerische Museum für Volkskunde Basel.

Katalog: Musikhistorisches Museum von Wilhelm Heyer in Cöln. Katalog v. Georg Kinsky. Hrsg. v. Wilh. Heyer. Bd. 2: Zupf- und Streichinstrumente. Köln, Kommissions-Verlag v. Breitkopf & Härtel, 1912.

Katalog: Steiermärkisches Landesmuseum Joanneum. Steirisches Volkskundemuseum, Außenstelle Stainz. Katalog Nr. 6: Holz, Naturformen. Kat. u. Ausst.: Maria Kundegraber u. Dieter Weiss. Schloß Stainz, 1981. 52 S., Bildtaf.

Katalog: Studentisches Brauchtum. Ausstellung 20. Mai bis 3. Juli 1983. Niederösterreichisches Landesmuseum – volkskundliche Sammlung. Österr. Verein f. Studentengeschichte. = Katalog des NÖ Landesmuseums, Neue Folge Nr. 138, Wien 1983.

Klever, Ulrich: Der Stock als Waffe. Stockfechten u. Selbstverteidigung mit dem Stock. In: Der Stocksammler, H. 4/1983.

Klever, Ulrich: Stöcke. Originalausg. Mit 152 Abb., München, Heyne, 1980. 142 S. = Heyne Sammlerbibliothek, Bd. 9.

Knoppe, Hugo: Handbuch der Drechslerei. Mit 343 Abb., Leipzig, Steiger, 1938.

Köllman, Erich: Berliner Porzellan. Bd. 1 u. 2. Braunschweig, Klinkhardt & Biermann, 1963.

Krünitz, Johann Georg (Hrsg.): Ökonomisch-technologische Encyclopädie. T. 156. Berlin, 1832.

La Salle, J.-B. de: Les règles de la bienséance et de la civilité chrétienne divisées en deux parties. Lille, Lefort, 1840.

Lind, Karl: Ueber den Krummstab. Eine archäologische Skizze. Wien, Prandel u. Ewald, 1863. 55 S.

Manga, János: Herdsmen's Art in Hungary. 2nd ed. Corvinia Verlag, 1972. 86 S., Taf. = Hungarian Folk Art 5.

Meyer, H. C.: H. C. Meyer Jr. Kommanditgesellschaft auf Aktien. Hamburg-Harburg/Elbe. 1818–1918. Harburg, Bertram, 1918. 30 S., Abb.

Moeck, Hermann: Spazierstockinstrumente und Czakane, englische und wiener Flageolette. In: Studia istrumentorum musicae popularis III, S. 149–151 u. 152–163. Abb. = Musikhistoriska museets skrifter 5. Stockholm, Musikförlaget NMS 6523 Musikhistoriska museet, 1974.

Moeller, Ernst von: Die Rechtssitte des Stabbrechens. In: Zeitschrift der Savigny-Stiftung für Rechtsgeschichte, Bd. 21, S. 27. Weimar, 1900.

Monek, Francis H.: Canes. In: The Encyclopedia of Collectibles. Alexandria/Virg., Time-Life Books C., 1978. S. 42–53, Abb.

Nachricht: Zuverlässige Nachricht von der Lebensart auf der Universität Göttingen. Eine Werbeschrift aus dem Jahre 1739.

Neuenhoff, G.: Ein Ziegenhainer-Stock. In: Einst und Jetzt. Bd. 27. Jahrbuch 1982 des Vereins für corpsstudentische Geschichtsforschung.

Philippovich, Eugen von: Elfenbein. Ein Handbuch f. Sammler u. Liebhaber. 2., neubearb. u. stark erw. Aufl. München, Klinkhardt & Biermann, 1982. 480 S. = Bibliothek für Kunst- u. Antiquitätenfreunde, Bd. XVII.

Pinto, Edward H.: Treen and other wooden bygones. An encyclopedia and social history. London, Bell & Sons, 1969. X, 458 S., Abb.

Reichs-Adressbuch für die gesamte Schirm- und Stockbranche. I. Ausg. Dresden, Verlag J. Fesq, 1929.

Ritz, J. M.: Stock und Stab. In: Jahrbuch 1937 des Bayerischen Landesvereins für Heimatschutz – hrsg. in Verbindung mit dem Bayer. Landesamt f. Denkmalpflege u. dem Bayer. Nationalmuseum.

Schild, Wolfgang: Alte Gerichtsbarkeit. Vom Gottesurteil bis zum Beginn der modernen Rechtsprechung. München, Callwey Verlag, 1980.

Schirm u. Stock. Fachblatt für die gesamte Schirm- u. Stockindustrie Deutschlands und des Auslands. Offizielles Organ des Verbandes Deutscher Schirmspezial-Geschäfte. Dresden, Verlag J. Fesq, 1915ff.

Schlumberger, Eveline: Cannes à Coups, Cannes à Rêves. Secrètement armé ou précieusement orné, ce support de la main l'est aussi de l'imagination: à preuve ces quelques cannes d'une importante collection privée. In: Connaissance des Arts, No. 339, Mai 1980, S. 74–79.

Schneider-Henn, Dietrich: Nicht ohne Stock durch die Landschaft. In: Antiquitäten-Zeitung, Nr. 8, 1983.

Schönberger, Guido: Narwal-Einhorn. Studien über einen seltenen Werkstoff. Städel-Jahrbuch 1935/36, S. 167–247, Abb.

Schuhmann, Helmut: Der Scharfrichter. Kempten, 1964.

Sedlmayr, Fritz: Die Geschichte der Spatenbrauerei unter Gabriel Sedlmayr dem Älteren und dem Jüngeren 1807–1874 sowie Beiträge zur bayerischen Brauereigeschichte dieser Zeit. Teil I u. II – I. Teil: München, Kommissionsverlag v. Piloty & Loehle, 1934. VIII, 362 S., Taf. – II. Teil: 1840–1874. Nürnberg, Carl, 1951. 467 S., Taf.

Seitz, Heribert: Blankwaffen I. Ein waffenhist. Handbuch. Braunschweig, Klinkhardt & Biermann, 1965. XII, 445 S., 318 Abb., 15 Farbtaf. = Bibliothek für Kunst- u. Antiquitätenfreunde, Bd. IV.

Senger, Daniel: Von der Ärztetracht zum »Gott in Weiß«. In: Schwarzhaupt-Journal.

Stein, Kurt: Canes & Walking Sticks. York/Pennsyl., Liberty Cap Books, 1974, 175 S., Abb.

Steinbeis, Dr. von: Referat des X. Ausschusses über Holzwaren und kurze Waren verschiedener Art. In: Bericht der Beurtheilungs-Commission bei der allgemeinen deutschen Industrie-Ausstellung zu München 1854. 10. Heft. München, Franz, 1855.

Stengel, Walter: Guckkasten Altberliner Curiosa. Berlin, 1962.

Stock–Pfeife–Schirm. Organ für die Fachgruppe der Ladeninhaber, sowie für die Horn-, Elfenbein-, Bernstein- u. Schildpattwaren-Branche im Reichsverband für das selbständige deutsche Drechsler-Gewerbe E. V. Beilage zur »Deutschen Drechsler-Zeitung«. Leipzig-Gohlis, Verlag F. E. Steiger, 1926 ff.

Sturtevant, Erich: Vom guten Ton im Wandel der Jahrhunderte. Mit e. Kostümtaf. Die Entwicklung der modischen Trachten von 1200 bis 1850. Berlin u. a., Dt. Verlagshaus Bong & Co., 1917. VIII, 368 S.

Supplejack, Solomon: Hints to the Bearers of Walking Sticks and Umbrellas. 2nd ed. London, Murray u. a., 1808. 31 S.

Tegner, Bruce: Stick Fighting: Self-Defense. Ventura/Calif., Thor Publ. Co., 1973. 127 S., Abb.

Thiel, Erika: Geschichte des Kostüms. Die europ. Mode v. d. Anfängen bis zur Gegenwart. Berlin, Henschelverlag Kunst u. Gesellschaft, 1968. Taf. u. Abb.

Verebélyi, Kincso: Ungarische Hirtenstäbe. In: Volkskunst. Zeitschrift für volkstümliche Sachkultur, H. 3, Aug. 1983, S. 150–154. München, Callwey Verlag, 1983.

Vorbrodt, Günter W. u. Ingeburg: Die akademischen Szepter und Stäbe in Europa. Vorgelegt am 14. Juni 1969 v. Walter Paatz. Heidelberg, Carl Winter, 1971.

Walking Sticks: Where Walking Sticks Grow. In: Answers, June 24th 1893, S. 84.

Waugh, Norah: The Cut of Men's Clothes 1600–1900. London, Faber and Faber LTD., 1964. 160 S.

Weigand, Wilhelm (Hrsg.): Der Hof Ludwigs XIV. Nach den Denkwürdigkeiten des Herzogs von Saint-Simon. Hrsg. u. eingel. v. Wilh. Weigand. 3., verm. Aufl. Leipzig, Insel-Verlag, 1925. 525 S., Abb.

Weinhold, Karl: Über die Bedeutung des Haselstrauches im altgermanischen Kultus und Zauberwesen. In: Zeitschrift des Vereins für Volkskunde. Hrsg. v. Karl Weinhold. Jg. 11, Berlin, 1901.

Weiß, Eugen: Die Entdeckung des Volks der Zimmerleute. Zünftiges von Zimmerleuten: ihr Leben und Fühlen, erhaltenes Brauchtum, Redensarten in Schwaben, Mären, Ränke und Schwänke, Sprüche und Flüche, Neckereien, Rammlieder, Zimmer- und Schnursprüche, Handwerkslieder. Jena, Diederichs, 1923.

Wiegersma, H.: Volkskunst in de Nederlanden. Klein-Beeldhouwwerk, Boekdrukkerij »Helmond«, 1941.

Winant, Lewis: Firearms Curiosa. London, Arco Publ. LTD., 1956.

Photo Credits

Y.W. Kadri made 221 photographs for this book

The others are form: Bavarian Administration of Federal castles, parks and lakes (3); Christie's (4); C. Dike (2); Dumoulin (1); Esbola (72), General administration of the Former Ruling Prussian Royal House, Hero Bild (1); M. German (15); German Museum (1); R. Guillemot (2); J. Hartz (10); Auction house Ineichen (2); U. Klever (8); Le Louvre des Antiquaires (2); St. Moses (2), Sotheby's (9); Federal Institute for Musical research, Foundation Prussian Cultural Heritage (3)

Fig 52 was made by Christel Aumann, Munich. All other text illustrations are from the author's archives

Values are provided for the photo illustrations (1-344). Values vary immensely according to the condition of the piece, the location of the market, and the overall quality of the design and manufacture. Condition is always of paramount importance in assigning value. The values in this guide reflect fair market value. Values vary by geographic location and those at specialty antique shows will vary from those at general shows. And, of course, being in the right place at the right time may make all the difference.

All these factors make it impossible to create an absolutely accurate reference, but we can offer a guide. The gadget and weapons canes are avidly sought after and are very volatile in price; some are also very rare.

The prices are listed in order of photo illustration number. "N.A." is used when a value is unavailable for a particular cane. No values are assigned to photos illustrating cane woods or other groupings. The estimated value ranges are in U.S. dollars.

Illustration number is followed by dollar value.

Value Reference

1 .... Rare	41 .... Rare	1000-1200;
2 .... Rare	42 600-900	1000-1200;
3 1500-2000	43 600-900	600-800;
4 2000-2400	44 250-500	600-800;
5 .... N.A.	45 600-900	1200-1800
6, 7 .... N.A.	46 150-250	77 .... left: 1800-2800;
8 .... 1100-1200 ea.	47 250-450	right: 1500-2500
9 1200-1300	48 1500-2000	79 250-500
10 1100-1200	49, 50 .... 600-800 ea.	80 .... N.A.
11 .... N.A.	51 200-400	81 400-600
12 .... Rare	52 300-500	82, 83 .... Rare
13 1000-1500	53 600-800	84 200-400
14 800-1200	54 800-1000	85-87 600-800
15 .... 600-1000 ea.	55 50-150	88, 89 600-800
16 800-1200	56 .... 400-600 ea.	90 400-600
17 800-1200	57 .... 400-600 ea.	91 .... 600-900 ea.
18 800-1200	58 700-900	92 400-600
19 .... 600-800 ea.	61 150-250	93 550-650
20-22 .... 600-800 ea.	62 250-500	94 400-600
24 1500-2000	63 .... N.A.	95 400-500
25 .... Rare	64 .... N.A.	96 150-250
26 400-600	65 600-700	97 300-500
27, 28 .... N.A.	66 700-800	98 600-800
29 800-1000	67 400-600	99, 100 1200-1500
30 500-700	68 500-700	101 1200-1500
31 1500-2000	69 .... 300-500 ea.	102 500-700
32 600-900	70, 71 450-650	103, 104 .... 800-900 ea.
33 1500-2500	72, 73 450-650	105 500-700
34 1500-2500	74 450-650	106 500-700
35 .... N.A.	75 450-650	107, 108 250-450
36 .... N.A.	76 .... left to right:	109 525-625
37 300-500	600-900;	110 550-650
38 .... N.A.	600-800;	111, 112 .... 100-200 ea.
39, 40 800-1000	600-900;	113 200-400

114-116 125-225	192 700-900	258 600-750
117, 118 .... 150-250 ea.	193 600-800	259 300-400
119 200-400	194 400-600	260-264 .... Rare
120 200-400	195 400-600	265 600-750
121 200-400	196 600-800	266 600-750
122 300-500	197 375-575	267 450-600
124 1500-2500	198 500-700	268 450-600
125 500-650	199 600-800	269 300-500
126 500-650	200 600-800	270 600-800
127 650-800	201 500-700	271 9000-12000
128, 129 2000-2500	202 400-600	272 .... Rare
130 .... N.A.	203 .... right: 1500-2500	273 .... Rare
131 550-750	204 800-1200	274 .... Rare
132 600-800	205 800-1200	275 .... Rare
133 1300-1800	206 400-600	276 .... Rare
134 1000-1800	207 400-600	277 700-900
135 650-800	208 800-1200	278 .... N.A.
136, 137 1000-1800	209 .... N.A.	279 .... Rare
138 .... N.A.	210 .... N.A.	280-282 .... 150-350 ea.
139 800-1200	211 .... N.A.	283 600-750
140 .... N.A.	212 600-800	284 400-600
141, 142 .... Rare	213 800-1200	285 400-600
143 800-1200	214 1000-1300	286 600-750
144, 145 1200-1800	215 900-1300	287 .... Rare
146, 147 800-1200	216 900-1300	288 800-1200
148, 149 800-1200	217 800-1000	289 800-1200
150, 151 800-1200	218, 219 600-750	290 .... N.A.
152, 153 800-1200	220 .... N.A.	291 2000-3000
154, 155 650-800	221 .... Rare	292 750-1000
156, 157 800-1200	222 1600-2200	293, 294 .... Rare
158 500-700	223 1000-1500	295, 296 .... Rare
159 500-700	224 600-800	297 .... Rare
160 400-600	225 1000-3000	298, 299, 301 700-1000
161 .... N.A.	226 600-800	300 700-1000
162 1000-1500	227 400-600	304 600-900
163 800-1200	228 600-800	305 600-900
164 400-600	229 .... N.A.	306 600-900
165 700-900	230 .... N.A.	307, 308 .... N.A.
166 700-900	231 .... Rare	309 .... Rare
167 700-900	232 .... N.A.	310 600-800
168 800-1200	233 1000-1500	311 .... Rare
169 .... N.A.	234 600-800	312 1000-1500
170 1500-2500	235 200-400	314, 315 850-1200
171 1000-1500	236 100-300	316, 317 850-1200
172 1000-1500	237 100-300	318 2000-3000
173 .... Rare	238 100-200	321 .... N.A.
174 200-400	239 300-500	322 700-900
175 .... N.A.	240 .... 50-150 ea.	323 .... 300-600 ea.
176 400-600	241 500-700	324, 325 1500-2500
177 400-600	242 200-400	326 1500-2500
178 400-600	243 450-650	327, 328 ...... 750-1000 ea.
179 400-600	244 350-400	329 .... N.A.
180 400-600	245 400-600	330 700-900
181 800-1200	246 .... N.A.	331 500-700
182 600-800	247 600-750	332 500-700
183 600-800	248 .... N.A.	333 .... N.A.
184 600-800	249 .... N.A.	334 350-500
185 800-1200	250 600-750	335 350-500
186 2000-3000	251 600-750	336 350-500
187 400-600	252 600-750	337 800-1200
188 600-800	253 650-750	338 800-1200
189 700-900	254, 255 750-1000	339 800-1200
190 .... 600-800 (reg. size)	256 300-400	340, 341 500-700
191 600-800	257 300-400	342-344 750-1000

Index

Numbers in plain text refer to pages, bold numbers to illustration numbers